Praise for Coping with Cancer

"This book is absolutely fantastic—it will be so very impactful and helpful. I am thrilled to have this widely available."

—WILLIAM S. BREITBART, MD, Jimmie C. Holland Chair in Psychiatric Oncology; Chairman, Department of Psychiatry and Behavioral Sciences, Memorial Sloan Kettering Cancer Center

"I will always remember the exact moment I received my first diagnosis of breast cancer, as well as my second diagnosis 15 years later. Over the years, I have nourished myself emotionally and intellectually by reading books on the challenges of living with cancer. None has had a greater impact than *Coping with Cancer*. This book is a treasure trove of tools and skill sets that can be life changing as you navigate the road ahead. It is beautifully written in a personal, authentic, totally relatable voice. It holds a special place on my shelf—as I predict it will on yours!"

—DEBBIE L., New York City

"In my 30-plus years as an oncology social worker, many books on living with cancer have crossed my desk. Books on this topic tend to be based on either personal experience or professional know-how; this guide is an excellent combination of the two and perfect to help you feel more in control and manage the uncertainty of living with a cancer diagnosis."

—SARA GOLDBERGER, MSSW, ACSW, LCSW-R, cancer survivor and President, Association of Oncology Social Workers

"I am deeply grateful to the authors for this respectful, compassionate, very practical guide. There was nothing like this book when my mother was diagnosed with cancer in 1954, back when people would not even say 'the C-word.' In fact, there has been nothing like it until now! As the survivor of two aggressive cancers myself, I wish I had had this book when I was diagnosed. The authors provide a manageable, step-wise approach to coping with an individual and interpersonal disaster. They draw on knowledge from both DBT and psychoanalysis to produce a welcome, creative synthesis."

—NANCY MCWILLIAMS, PhD, ABPP, Graduate School of Applied and Professional Psychology, Rutgers, The State University of New Jersey

"An important book for us all to read. It is practical, actionable, down to earth, and wise."

—REV. JOAN HALIFAX, Abbot, Upaya Zen Center, and author of *Standing at the Edge*

"This book is filled with Stuntz's wisdom from her years sharing Linehan's skills with cancer patients, and her personal experience of facing cancer skillfully. It offers thoughtful, practical, and heartfelt guidance for managing emotional distress, communicating needs, and finding meaning. As a DBT clinician and cancer survivor/fighter myself, I rely on the skills in this book to face my diagnosis, treatments, and uncertainties, and to continue engaging in my personal and professional life. This book is an invaluable resource for patients, loved ones, and support groups facing the emotional rollercoaster of a cancer diagnosis."

—SETH AXELROD, PhD, Director of DBT Services and Associate Professor of Psychiatry, Yale–New Haven Psychiatric Hospital

COPING WITH CANCER

COPING with CANCER

*DBT Skills to Manage Your Emotions—
and Balance Uncertainty with Hope*

Elizabeth Cohn Stuntz, LCSW
Marsha M. Linehan, PhD

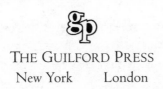

THE GUILFORD PRESS
New York   London

Copyright © 2021 Elizabeth Cohn Stuntz and Marsha M. Linehan

Published by The Guilford Press
A Division of Guilford Publications, Inc.
370 Seventh Avenue, Suite 1200, New York, NY 10001
www.guilford.com

The information in this volume is not intended as a substitute for
consultation with healthcare professionals. Each individual's health
concerns should be evaluated by a qualified professional.

Printed in the United States of America

Last digit is print number: 9   8   7   6   5   4   3   2   1

Library of Congress Cataloging-in-Publication Data is available from the
publisher.

ISBN 978-1-4625-4202-4 (paperback) — ISBN 978-1-4625-4505-6
(hardcover)

Contents

Acknowledgments

Elizabeth Cohn Stuntz

This book is a testimony to the power of connection and community. So many people supported and worked with me, read drafts, and provided feedback and constructive criticism.

It never would have happened without the spirit and brilliance of Marsha Linehan. My friend, mentor, and Zen teacher always had faith in me. She was open to my ideas even when they were very different from hers, offering a special balance of simultaneously challenging *and* encouraging me. Her lifelong commitment to helping as many people as possible was a guiding light that carried me forward.

My husband, Mike, provided a steadfast loving presence and immeasurable support throughout the writing process. Like Marsha, he both challenged and encouraged me through the ups and downs to keep my eye on my priority of helping others to manage life with cancer. With no background in DBT, he was a great reader, always helping me try to clarify my main point. He has reviewed so many drafts that he could probably now be certified to teach DBT!

I would like to recognize Gilda's Club Westchester and its dedicated staff for their innovative psychosocial support for individuals with cancer and their loved ones. In the earliest stages of offering DBT to people with cancer, I was privileged to work with Christine Consiglio, Miranda Dold, Erica Forest, Eric Kelly, Melissa Lang, Sarah Reynolds, and Stacy Weissberg.

Extra-special appreciation goes to my two very dear friends and colleagues Ronda Reitz and Joan Chess. Ronda provided invaluable assistance in most effectively communicating DBT. Joan read almost every single draft, offering very helpful feedback and support. During the years of writing, I was blessed with many other readers, including Debbie Chapin, Ellen Cohn, Carole Geithner, Sara Goldberger, Bill Hartman, Joan Macfarlane, Katherine Sailer, Brad Swanson, and Priscilla Warner. Thanks so much to Kitty Moore and Christine Benton at The Guilford Press for all their invaluable help and guidance.

Many others generously contributed their personal experience and/ or professional expertise, including Seth Axelrod, La Shaune Johnson, Ken Lerer, Eddie Marritz, Edythe Held Mencher, Robin Newman, Katie Stuntz, Alice Taranto, and Lisa Witten. Special thanks goes to the many unnamed individuals whose personal experiences with cancer are the basis of the stories shared in this book.

Those who went the extra mile to offer support and assistance include Perry D'Alba and the staff at D'Alba IT, Eric Brown, Elaine Franks, the Larchmont Public Library Reference Desk, and Geraldine Rodriguez. I am especially grateful to Ken Weinrib, who steadfastly guided me through the unforeseen complicated ups and downs of bringing this book to publication.

Finally, I would also like to acknowledge my own professional community, the Westchester Center for the Study of Psychoanalysis and Psychotherapy.

Marsha M. Linehan

My family has been a constant source of unconditional love and support in helping me make this book a reality. My dearest Geraldine, Nate, and Catalina lovingly fill my days with everything and anything needed to experience joy. The fact that my sister, Aline, lives on the other side of the country doesn't for a minute minimize her daily contact and support. My brothers, Earl, John, Marston, and Michael, are my reinforcement team.

When my Zen student Elizabeth Stuntz suggested we try to offer DBT skills to people living with cancer, my brother Marston's work at the National Cancer Institute inspired me to pursue the idea. I imagined that writing this book and applying my work to cancer patients would fulfill my promise of always finding a way to help others.

My beloved Zen teachers Willigis Jäger and Pat Hawke were crucial to my thinking about balancing acceptance and change and mindfully focusing on the present. I will always be thankful for their teachings and their wisdom. A special recognition goes to my Zen student and DBT practitioner Ronda Reitz, whose valuable contribution helped to shape the writing of this book. I am also very appreciative of her role, along with that of Randy Wolbert, in carrying forward my Zen mindfulness retreats.

My fabulous friends Ron and Marcia Baltrusis have played an extra-special role at this time. They have been not only a personal source of love and encouragement, sharing our spiritual community, but also an invaluable sounding board on cancer and DBT.

I am so appreciative of the continued support and friendship of my assistants Thao Truong and Elaine Franks, as well as my fabulous editor Kitty Moore at The Guilford Press. And to my colleagues and former students, thank you for taking DBT to people and places who need this treatment.

Introduction

"You have cancer!" I can still remember the exact moments I heard those jolting words applied to my mother, to other loved ones, and later to me. My mother used to call cancer "the Big C" so she didn't actually have to say the word. Could this word really now apply to you?

While you may feel alone, you are among 15.5 million Americans currently living with this illness. This news is one of the most difficult things you'll ever have to face. And now you have to figure out how to cope! Can you find a way to be hopeful without using all your energy trying to pretend you're not afraid? What can you do when you wake up with fear and dread and don't want to get out of bed? Is it possible to acknowledge feeling sad without being overwhelmed by emotion? How can you let others know what you want and need when you feel too vulnerable to ask?

Cancer treatment has a come a long way, and survival rates have risen steadily over the years. Yet even a reliable diagnosis, realistic prognosis, and the best available treatment that may save your life rarely tell you how to manage the emotional trauma. Experts agree that effective coping strategies are a crucial part of cancer treatment. Studies have shown that psychosocial support for cancer patients can often improve quality of life and survival rates. In spite of that, social and emotional treatment has not kept pace with the remarkable medical progress. This book attempts to bridge that gap.

A Groundbreaking Framework to Help You Cope: Dialectical Behavior Therapy

Dr. Marsha Linehan, named by *Time* magazine as one of the geniuses and visionaries whose work has transformed our world, developed dialectical behavior therapy (DBT) to help people cope when life feels intolerable. She created skills based on the wisdom of Zen and contemplative prayer among other traditions to help people survive the tragedies and challenges of life. Her skills have been proven effective in helping suicidal people tolerate unbearable situations, from major losses to the absence of meaning in life. Marsha, who lost her mother to cancer, has now collaborated with me (Elizabeth) to offer you these strategies to help you cope with a diagnosis that you may have never anticipated and would never choose.

I am a psychoanalyst with a family therapy background who has a long-standing personal and professional involvement in providing emotional support to people with cancer. The disease took my grandmother as a young woman and then cut my mother's life short. I also lost many cherished friends to cancer, and fears about my own health as well as possible implications for my treasured children always lurked in the back of my mind. Then came my own diagnosis. As Marsha's Zen student, trained to be open to all experiences and perspectives, I recognized the potential of the DBT framework for people living with cancer. I then saw the value of DBT firsthand after piloting the skills with many individuals and at a cancer support organization.

How DBT Can Help

Effective coping is not about the particular event or circumstances but how you react to what has happened—what you think, how you feel, and what you do. DBT offers you concrete skills to realistically assess whatever difficulty you are facing so you can decide what to do and what not to do. The skills include ways to manage your emotions, communicate with others, tolerate distress, and live meaningfully. At this overwhelming time it can be particularly valuable to know how to be clearer about what is happening and how you are feeling as well as to have tools to deal with the stress. When you have ways to cope with the wildly fluctuating emotions and runaway thoughts that can come with cancer, you may be more able to respond wisely to the threats without overreacting to the dangers and more effectively express your concerns to others.

These strategies can be useful wherever you are in your cancer experience—recently diagnosed, in the midst of treatment, posttreatment, in remission, or a long-term survivor. Although the book is written for people living with cancer, loved ones have effectively used the skills too.

The *D* of *DBT* stands for **dialectics,** a 50-cent word which means that **two things that seem to be opposite can both be true.** What does this have to do with cancer? When we are upset, it is easy to reduce life to one way *or* the other, simply seeing things as black *or* white, good *or* bad. Sometimes people minimize their problems *or* see their situation as a total disaster. Have you ever concluded that because you are no longer completely healthy, you are going to die? Do you think that you are powerless because you can't totally control everything that is happening in your life?

Balance is key to effective coping. Dialectics makes it clear that it is possible to think, feel, or act in more than just one way. You can be *both* unhappy that you have cancer *and* still be happy about parts of your life. It is possible to be frightened *and* have hope. You can feel weak *and* act strong. It is possible to feel helpless that you can't control everything that is happening *and* recognize that there are changes you can make. You can see that your feelings are understandable. You are coping the best way you know how right now *and* recognize that it is possible to learn more effective strategies.

Easier said than done! Constant change and the roller coaster of life with cancer can throw you off balance. **Life is always changing, and your moods may be as changeable as the weather.** At one moment the sun shines brightly. Later, clouds may drift by, casting a shadow on the brightness. Then a dark storm may arise. In the darkness, you may even forget the sun exists. Afterwards, different weather comes through. Perhaps the sun reappears. And at the end of the day, when the sun goes down, it is dark again.

Right now the weather may not be changing as quickly as you want and need. Yet, even if you can't control when and how the weather changes, you are not powerless. There are effective ways to get through the storm you are in at this moment. **You cope most effectively by choosing to stay**

open to other possibilities and viewpoints. In dark times, hope comes from remembering that light exists even when you can't see it. The skills in this book can show you how to change the ways you feel or think or what you do by balancing opposite emotions, thoughts, or actions.

What You Will Find in This Book

While many others are living with cancer, each individual's experience is unique. This book offers you ways to create your own customized set of coping strategies and help you find the wisdom to know when each skill might be effective for you. We encourage you to read the entire book, in order, as the skills build on each other.

Each chapter includes the voices and collective wisdom of people touched by cancer so you have an opportunity to connect with their experiences. To ensure confidentiality, the personal accounts are fictionalized composites of actual stories and typical responses. The remarks in quotations come from specific individuals and are used here with their permission. Some chapters also include exercises so you can practice the skills on your own. Although the book is the result of our collaboration, for ease of reading, it is written in my (Elizabeth's) first-person voice.

The first two chapters present ways to deal with a cancer diagnosis. Chapter 1 offers a framework to help you understand your response to diagnosis, see that your reactions are not unusual, and respond in a more balanced way than most of us are inclined to do. Chapter 2 presents tools to help you make effective decisions, including trusting the inherent wisdom within yourself. This chapter includes mindfulness skills, which can be an invaluable way to get a clearer, more complete and accurate picture of your situation.

Next we move into life with cancer, including how to cope with emotions and communicate with others. Chapter 3 offers concrete strategies you can use to manage your emotions, including the apprehension about living with a roller coaster of intense feelings and the worry about the impact of stress on cancer. Chapters 4–6 then delve into specific emotions—fear and anxiety, grief, and anger. Each of these chapters shows ways for you to recognize your feelings and gives you practical tools to cope with them.

Chapters 7 and 8 present strategies for communicating constructively with family, friends, colleagues, and medical providers. These chapters cover skills that will help you make your needs known while protecting relationships and your self-respect.

Chapter 9 focuses on sources of deeper meaning and comfort. As many look for sources of connection to something greater than themselves when they feel a threat to survival, a discussion of spirituality is included.

> *We can not change the cards we are dealt, just how we play the hand.*
> —RANDY PAUSCH

ONE

Dealing with the News That You Have Cancer

A cancer diagnosis can feel like an intruder just barged into your home. Reactions may range from unhappiness to devastation. For some, hearing the news is in itself a trauma. Sara, who trembled though she wasn't cold, compared the jolt to being struck by lightning. Suddenly her life was changed, now defined as BC and AC—before and after cancer.

All kinds of thoughts can come up. Sara said to herself:

This can't be happening!

I can't deal with this.

My life has no room for cancer.

I feel like my head is full of cotton candy! I can't think straight.

Could I actually die?

What did the doctor just say to me? I am not getting this right.

But I'm so healthy!

Am I overreacting? Stop panicking.

You're an emotional wreck. Get a grip on yourself.

This new territory may stir up unfamiliar, powerful emotions. Maybe you are shocked by your feelings or feel inundated by confusing emotions.

Perhaps you find yourself panicked, enraged by this twist of fate or frozen with fear you've never experienced before. Some feel desperate to do anything possible to stop those intense feelings.

I am uncomfortable when I remember some of my initial reactions. At first, I was numb and made a joke. I had no idea what I was actually feeling. I only knew I was determined to stay in control and not feel vulnerable. I believed any emotion would flood and overwhelm me. I thought:

> *I am a therapist. I have dealt with lots of people with cancer. I should be able to cope.*
>
> *Strong feelings will unnerve me and leave me out of control.*
>
> *If I feel weak and fragile, I might not have the strength to fight for my health.*
>
> *I am not going to be defenseless and helpless.*
>
> *I won't "allow myself" to be scared, sad, or frustrated.*
>
> *If I am gripped by grief and anxiety, I will turn into a terrified and depressed person.*
>
> *Worry won't rule me!*

There Is No Right or Wrong Way to Feel

On some level I wondered whether my reaction was strange. Another woman joked to her doctor that what she really needed most right now was a "mental hospital." It turns out we were not the only ones who worried about how we were handling our feelings. In a classic Memorial Sloan-Kettering study of patients' troubling symptoms, four out of the top five concerns of cancer patients were about their emotional reactions.

It is important to recognize that **no reaction is either unusual or wrong.** More than likely, others have felt as you do. The wide range of responses can run from feeling very emotional like Sara to my very controlled response. Some people are very conscious of their bodily responses, feelings, and thoughts. Others are totally unaware. Genes and personal history may shape your reaction. Previous emotional or medical difficulties can also be an influence.

Uncomfortable feelings can quickly turn into "I am bad"—deciding there is something wrong with you or your ways of coping. Many lose faith in their ability to manage or start blaming themselves. They may wonder, *Why me?* Sara became self-critical and decided she was an emotional wreck. Another person said, "The first night was terrible for me. I panicked. Who would take care of my kids? I realized quickly that I needed help and would have to lean on other people, something I had not done so well before. How did I miss this lump?"

It is going to be important for you to notice self-criticism and be kinder to yourself. Indeed, some people invalidate their own feelings. Like me, many turn away from how they *do* feel to how they believe they are supposed to feel. They may try to avoid certain emotions or look to the "rules" for guidance about how they *should* feel. Sara believed she was not supposed to be so sad and should be more upbeat. Are you telling yourself that you should be braver or calmer? Or that you should attend to business as usual or think of the people who depend on you first? Have you decided that you should "let it all out" or keep it to yourself? These *shoulds* are not helpful! They put harmful pressure on you to change your natural emotional reactions. The *shoulds* only distract you from what's most important: paying attention to how you really do feel and what you really want at this point in your life.

Tuning In to Whatever You Are Feeling and Thinking Is Key

Your emotions, thoughts, and physical sensations offer valuable information. They can tell you what's wrong and needs to be addressed as well as what's going right that should be pursued. There is no time when getting this valuable input is more crucial than when you have cancer. Yet there is no time when it's more difficult to take in a lot of new and unwelcome information than when you've just been diagnosed.

Consider what happens when an electrical circuit is overloaded. The circuit breaker shuts off your electricity, and your lights, appliances, computer, and everything else stop working. In the same way, when you feel overwhelmed, your capacity to deal with life can be strained. **Your coping circuit includes your emotions, thoughts, and physical sensations that work together and influence each other simultaneously and**

reciprocally. Just as you look at your circuit breakers to detect the problem with your electricity, it's going to be helpful for you to learn how to pay careful attention to your emotions, thoughts, and bodily sensations to restore your most effective functioning. Let's start by looking at emotions.

Emotions

While everyone is unique, fear, sadness, and anger are considered the most common emotional responses to a cancer diagnosis. Let's look at how understandable these emotions are when you have cancer.

Fear

The word *cancer* stirs up a threat of danger. If you think you are at risk, fear is a logical reaction because it urges you to take self-protective action. Anxiety is reasonable if you believe you are at risk of not living as long, or not having the quality of life you hoped or imagined. Sara decided she was an emotional wreck because she was so frightened. Yet her worry makes sense if she imagines that her future and her family's future are in jeopardy. I initially believed that fear would make me weak until I came to realize that emotions did not have to control or define me. When we discuss fear in Chapter 4, you will see that being frightened at this moment does not have to mean you are a fearful person.

Sadness

The word *cancer* suggests the threat of loss. Grief is reasonable if you think you will be harmed or have to give up something meaningful to you. Sadness is understandable if you have to accept that your life will not follow the course you expected or planned. Sorrow and anguish make sense if cancer will make you ill, unable to take part in treasured activities or care for your family. Sara was reluctant to admit the validity of her own sadness. I imagined that if I allowed myself to cry I would never stop. While you may be worried that you will be overwhelmed by grief, after reading this book you will more than likely come to understand that emotions actually ebb and flow.

Anger

The word *cancer* can bring to mind the threat of a limited life. If you think your days will not turn out as you hoped and planned, frustration and anger are understandable. Indignation makes sense if you believe that you've lost your physical health. Agitation is reasonable if you are sure that you can no longer participate in cherished activities or that important relationships might be compromised. Anger is useful when you need to protect yourself or fight an injustice. It is understandable that Sara may feel annoyed if her medical needs aren't addressed. While you may be frightened that your anger will consume you as I initially was, Chapter 6 offers ways to use your anger constructively without letting it harm your relationships.

Thoughts

Our thoughts are another part of the circuit that impacts our functioning—both how we feel and how we act. The emotions we just described make sense if all of your assumptions about your life with cancer are reliable. But what if they're not? What if your ideas aren't accurate? If you are making unconfirmed assumptions, you are not alone. Let's take a look at how that happens.

The Tales We Tell Ourselves: Fiction or Nonfiction?

An unexpected diagnosis that shatters a dream of a comfortable, predictable path in life can stir up fear and vulnerability. Faced with danger and uncertainty, the brain can create stories to attempt to explain the situation and restore a sense of predictability and control.

Sara's mind flooded with overwhelming thoughts that repeated in an endless loop:

Nothing will ever be the same.

I probably won't be able to work.

I am going to be weak and sick all the time.

Who will take care of my kids?

I'll be dependent and a burden.

I am letting my family down.

I should be more upbeat.

Am I going to die?

Are all of Sara's beliefs true? Have her assumptions been verified by facts? Her apprehensive thoughts are understandable if she believes her illness puts her family's future in financial jeopardy. On the other hand, is she making herself more anxious by assuming she won't be able to work now when she doesn't know whether that's true? Mourning makes sense if she is going to die right away. But is she grieving the end of her life before she knows if she may be facing a period of treatment with a probability of return to normal functioning? Are unproven swirling ideas leaving her more frightened, sad, or angry than necessary?

Predicting the Worst by Getting Ahead of Yourself

It can be tricky to tell the difference between the realities of our situation and unconfirmed theories that are reactions to fear or anxiety. Both fear and anxiety stimulate ideas for responding to danger, but there is an important distinction that is valuable to understand. With **fear,** whether you have cancer or not, thoughts are based on a reaction to **present** actual danger. Right now. The fact is a hungry lion is in front of you. Fear mobilizes thoughts for immediate action. You run!

Anxiety, on the other hand, is about the **future.** Anxiety mobilizes thoughts to prepare you for something that *might* happen. There is a tendency to make assumptions that *may or may not* be factual. Anxiety prepares you for action that *may or may not* be necessary or productive.

It makes sense that when Sara is facing an operation, frightening ideas go through her mind as she is being wheeled into surgery. Some of her thoughts may even be constructive if, for example, she decides she is going to do everything possible to take good care of herself. At other moments, Sara, like all of us, may get ahead of herself and magnify the danger by telling herself stories about what *might* happen in the future.

Perhaps Sara is adding to her concerns by needlessly believing things that make her even more anxious. My coauthor, Marsha, refers to exaggerating harm as "catastrophizing." Plans or actions based on unproven ideas may not be constructive. Inaccurate dire assumptions may even leave us vulnerable to withdrawing from joyful parts of life or clinging to misleading promises of cure or remission. Imagine the cost to Sara and her family if she regards her ideas that she is a dependent burden who is letting her family down as facts and tries to protect them by keeping her distance.

Physical Sensations

Now let's look at the role of your physical sensations in the circuit. The human body and mind were designed to optimize functioning in prehistoric times—primarily to ensure self-preservation. The body innately scans to assess the safety of a situation. The nervous system responds to the apparent threat by telling our bodies to fight, take flight, or freeze. When the caveman saw the lion in front of him, his heart rate increased, his palms began to sweat, and his muscles tensed to prepare him to take action. He was terrified and ran. In this case, his physical reactions, emotions, and thoughts all worked together to create an effective response.

As we humans have evolved, this valuable innate fight-flight-or-freeze system for assessing risk may now also fuel anxiety. Modern-day men and women not only think but also ponder and ruminate, and our bodies respond the same way to anxiety as they do to fear.

The Negative Feedback Loop

Your body, thoughts, and emotions can get caught in an endless and unconstructive cycle. Whether or not the thoughts are factual, or the threat is real, your heart will beat faster and your stomach will be in knots in response to negative ideas about what *might* happen in the future. Your body will continue to believe there is an ongoing present threat. Your nervous system will be overloaded and send a continuous "UH-OH, DANGER!" message to fight, take flight, or freeze. Bathed in stress, your body will create chronic muscle tension as armor to prepare for danger.

This signal will fuel your anxiety, which in turn will increase your apprehensive thoughts. Those anxious ideas will feed your feelings of worry and nervousness.

Neuroscientists have also discovered that in scanning for threats, the mind has a biological bias toward the negative. Prehistoric humans could not afford to mistake a venomous snake for a stick. The Stone Age mind was predisposed to see something shaped like a snake and think. "My life is in danger. I better get out of here." As the brain is like Velcro for negative thoughts and Teflon for positive ones, assumptions can drift away from fact and predict a bleak future.

Imagine if the caveman continued to have negative thoughts even after escaping the snake.

Could that snake end up in my cave?

Maybe there are other dangerous animals that will come after me. I know there are lions out there too!

Maybe I should never leave my cave again!

As happens for the anxious caveman, your physical reactions, thoughts, and emotions can get stuck in an ongoing negative feedback loop. Just as the caveman's anxiety could cue him to panic even when he was looking at a stick on the ground, your negative feedback loop might throw you off balance, cuing you to treat your cancer diagnosis as a sure death sentence before you know the facts. If the caveman never leaves his cave again, he will surely die of starvation. If Sara takes her presumption of letting down her family as fact and keeps her distance, she risks denying herself and her loved ones a treasured and nourishing sense of love, support, and connection.

When you pay careful attention to the interplay between your emotions, your thoughts, and your body, you have the chance to understand your response and see where effective coping may be short-circuited and bring yourself back into balance. You can have a clearer picture of whether your emotions are hijacking your thoughts or you are making assumptions that stimulate a negative feedback loop, causing unproductive worry. This information can serve as a valuable guide to any changes you can make to manage more effectively.

Finding Balance through Dialectical Strategies

At times, the stories we tell ourselves are framed in a black-or-white, either/or way, and we can overreact or underestimate the problem. Dialectical strategies can help you find a more balanced approach to coping by keeping the opposite of your feelings, thoughts, and sensations in mind. Remember, things are not simply one way *or* the other. You can feel and think in two seemingly contradictory ways. You can be *both* worried *and* still have hope. It is possible to face what is happening *and* change the way you cope.

You may be able to see a new and more complete picture if you can keep opposing feelings and thoughts in mind. This balanced perspective may help you recognize that although you may not be 100% healthy, you're not necessarily going to die either. A 60% percent survival rate can be viewed as a catastrophe. On the other hand the odds are more favorable than not, but not worry free. A balanced middle perspective helps you *both* face that a cure is not a sure thing *and* recognize that the survival rate does include a reason for hope.

Wise Mind: A Balanced Middle Place

I wish I had understood that I could *both* accept how I was feeling *and* recognize that change was possible when I was diagnosed. I viewed my feelings in a very black-*or*-white way. I was desperately trying to minimize strong emotions. I believed I had to be calm, strong, and dispassionate *or* I would be weak and out of control. I was in what DBT calls **reasonable mind,** where thinking is extremely cool-headed and rational.

Sara was on the other extreme. She was in **emotion mind,** where feelings dominate thinking. In emotion mind, thinking is extremely hot, ruled by moods and feelings. In emotion mind you minimize facts, reason, and logic. In emotion mind you can overemphasize your worry about cancer and do not pay sufficient attention to hopeful information.

Your coping is most effective when your emotions and logic are in balance. Dialectical strategies help you **bring together opposites and find the balanced middle place between them**. The middle ground between the extremes of emotional and logical thinking is your **wise mind,** the overlapping center between emotion mind and reasonable mind.

States of Mind: Wise Mind

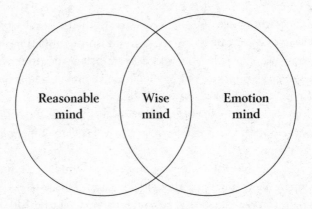

From *DBT Skills Training Handouts and Worksheets* (2nd ed.) by Marsha M. Linehan. Copyright © 2015 Marsha M. Linehan. Reprinted by permission of the author.

Wise mind takes a fuller view, respecting the value of reason *and* emotion, taking *both* logic and feelings into account. This third state of mind brings together left-brain rational thinking and right-brain emotion. In wise mind, you flexibly express emotions to cope more effectively. With a balanced wise mind perspective, you are less likely to panic and more likely to consider all potential paths toward health. In Chapter 2 we present ways to help you find and use your wise mind to make effective decisions.

Constantly Changing Perspectives to Come Closer to a Balanced Middle

Sara and I had to learn that fragility and fear were just one part of our stories—only one portion of the full picture. To get the **whole story,** we had to learn to **also pay attention to the opposite side** of the narrative that we were leaving out. We needed to also notice our strength, hope, and resilience.

There is an ongoing ebb and flow between the opposite sides, like playing on a seesaw, in which you constantly go back and forth. To make this balancing act work and move toward change, we had to pay attention to all aspects of our stories and acknowledge the other end of our seesaw. I risked being trapped on one end by denying strong emotions. I had to acknowledge my vulnerable emotions and beliefs without forgetting my resilience. Sara had to notice her strength and resilience so she would not be stuck on the frightened, vulnerable side.

Dinesh, now 28, described his balance between hope and fear when he had cancer at age 18: "I sometimes wondered why I wasn't more afraid. Some nights, after what felt like gallons of chemotherapy, I could barely sleep. . . . The next morning . . . my hopes for my future—not just the fear I wouldn't have one—made it possible to go back to the hospital. If I'd focused only on my fear, I wouldn't have been able to see past my nose."

It is important to realize that we shift back and forth from one side of the narrative to the other. When Sara gets up in the morning, she may instantly feel engulfed by fear that she won't get through cancer (thank you, negative bias!). But as she's standing in her kitchen drinking her first cup of coffee, she begins to feel alive and hopeful. An hour later she gets a call from her daughter from across the country, and the thought that she may not be able to function as the strong, supportive mom throughout her treatment makes her feel fragile and vulnerable. Then, on her walk with friends around the neighborhood, their shared stories and laughter make her feel connected to the world and to hope. And so it goes.

You start on one side of the seesaw. In order to avoid being stuck on one end and successfully push off to move, you need to be aware of the other extreme. Sara can be energized by the companionship of her friends even though her fear of needing a lot of help in the coming months lingers in her mind. As the two sides are connected, the weight on the opposite side affects how much force is needed to get going. When Sara is feeling particularly alone, weak, and blue, she may need to put even more effort into reminding herself that strength, resilience, and positive parts of life are part of her fullest story. At these points, an extra push from her friends might be especially helpful as well! This awareness of the continual movement between seemingly opposite sides helps to maintain a balanced middle ground.

Touchstones for Remembering That Change Is Possible

Hope is being able to see that there is light despite the darkness.
—DESMOND TUTU

In your darkest moments it is easier to find hope when you remember that you can choose to rebalance by also considering the other side of your fear or despair. It can be very useful to know what sounds, sensations, or images can be touchstones to keep the possibility of change in mind. For you, it may be a special memory or photo. Perhaps it is the shades of orange in the sky before sunrise or the soft touch of a pussywillow before the blossom of spring. Is it hearing the cry or feeling the soft touch of a new baby's skin? These touchstones are very personal. Maybe you are more open to new possibilities when you hear the opening chords of a special piece of music, even "Here Comes the Bride" or "Pomp and Circumstance."

Whatever or whoever helps you consider another perspective is valuable. The idea that your thoughts and feelings have another side can be very empowering. It is less threatening to accept fragility when you know that the complete picture includes strength. Catastrophic reactions can be less overwhelming when you realize there are inevitable ebbs and flows of your living seesaw. You do not have to be stuck in despair. A sense of hopelessness does not have to be a permanent state.

While none of us can know what will happen in our future, we want to hold on to light in the presence of darkness so we can make the most of the lives we actually have. If you keep the seesaw in motion, you can push off from that fearful end to reclaim hope on the other side. Your powerless reaction can be a springboard to action, to the possibility of change, to new ways to cope and to live the rest of your days as fully and meaningfully connected to who and what is most important to you as you can.

Let's now look at ways you can use your balanced wise mind to make effective decisions.

Two

How to Make Effective Decisions

Give me a break! Even before the shock of diagnosis has worn off, there are crucial decisions to be made.

Do I trust this diagnosis?

Is this proposed treatment the best choice?

Is my medical provider right for me?

Do I want a second opinion?

Is receiving one clear medical recommendation reassuring to you? Or do you want to know all the options? Perhaps you believe the only consideration is whatever recommendation comes with the best chance of survival. Are you worrying that your doctor will be offended if you want to think through your choice with family, friends, or other professionals?

Whatever your situation, constructive choices require you to take in and assess reliable information with your emotion and logic in balance. Yet when you've been thrown off by distressing news, it may be harder to hear and understand complex information. You may be more likely to miss crucial facts. Pausing to notice what is happening in and around you right now can help ensure your decisions are based on more complete and reliable information. This chapter introduces a strategy that will help you stop and pay attention to both the facts of the situation and your reactions: **mindfulness.** And, although you might not realize it, you already have the inherent intuition to make constructive choices—your wise mind. Let's begin by understanding the way wise mind (introduced in Chapter 1) helps with decision making.

Wise Mind

Wise mind is the **inherent wisdom that is a part of each of us, including you.** It's easy to assume other folks have this inner wisdom and you don't. This intuitive sense, what you "know to be true," is an invaluable guide to wise choices. It is the balanced middle of a seesaw informed by facts on one end *and* feelings on the other. You see the fullest story and get to the heart of the matter because you take both sides into consideration. Just as you can't stay in the balanced center of the seesaw, no one is in wise mind all the time. Yet with practice your balance improves.

The important thing to remember is you have wise mind even when you're not aware of it. Just as you don't always notice your breath or your beating heart, your wise mind is there even when you doubt it. It may not always be easy to find. Emotion mind and reasonable mind can get in the way. You may need to learn to dig deep to access your inner wisdom, so we include exercises to help you find your wise mind at the end of this chapter.

Wise Choices

The most effective decisions are made in wise mind with **balanced input from your feelings and your logic.** Beware of allowing your feelings to dominate a decision. When you are very emotional, your feelings can masquerade as the truth. You may "feel" something to be the case and have the urge to act right away. On the other hand, when you're overly rational, you may put on the brakes too tightly and miss valuable input from your feelings. Emotions can help you be in touch with your wishes, desires, beliefs and values. You don't want to overlook what is most important to you.

Wise mind is the balanced place of neither pushing forward nor holding back. It is the choice that still feels wise after you have paused and are calm. Wise decisions balance your subjective intuition with objective facts. You can listen to your doctor's valuable input without totally disregarding your own quality-of-life concerns. Recommendations based on medical facts are guides to inform, not rule, your choice. A wise decision is based on the whole picture, including everything you feel and value *and* what is factually true. It's important to remember that even when you are unsure about a choice, you have a wise mind.

Let's now explore a way to get a fuller and more reliable view of the current situation.

Mindfulness

We define mindfulness as:

Intentionally paying attention to the reality

at the present moment

without adding unproven assumptions or judgments

Let's break down the definition.

Paying Attention

In the ordinary course of events, it may not seem necessary to focus on being aware of all the details of your experience. Yet you may be astounded to see the information that can be overlooked when you aren't paying full attention. Consider checking out a fun YouTube video of a selective attention test at *www.youtube.com/watch?v=vJG698U2Mvo*.

If it's easy to miss information in the normal course of events, think about how much harder it can be when we are upset. Have you ever felt you were not taking in everything your doctor was saying to you? Emotions can color what we hear. When we are feeling overwhelmed, our attention can be pulled in many different directions. I was amazed to realize that the nine people listening to my mother's poor prognosis heard somewhat different versions of what we were told. Whether or not we are aware of it, we can sometimes cover our eyes and/or ears in painful situations. Who wants to see or hear a distressing reality? A woman who had multiple surgeries throughout her body liked to say, "My mirror does not exist below my neck."

Are you running from the fact that you have been told you have cancer or that a particular treatment is needed? Perhaps you are **confusing a fight for your health with a fight against facing the facts.** At times we may avoid the truth if we believe the myth that accepting the facts means we are passively giving in or that we want, like, or approve of the circumstances. It is important to keep in mind that it is possible to *both* acknowledge a painful reality *and* work aggressively to make changes.

Mindfulness has been described as "clearing the fog from the windshield" or shining a light on the circuit breakers to see which circuits are tripped. Marsha compares it to taking off a blindfold when you're walking through a room full of furniture. With the blindfold on, you remain in shutdown mode. You can miss important information and not have a full or realistic picture of what is in front of you. **When you are mindful, you deliberately choose to use all of your senses to notice the reality of what is happening at this moment.** You are no longer in the dark, vulnerable to stumbling blocks you hadn't noticed. Knowing the obstacles you have to navigate can help inform constructive choices.

The Present Moment

Long before mindfulness was in its current vogue, my mother's wise doctor used to warn her about unproductive conclusions she was prone to make when she got ahead of herself. His favorite saying was "Inch by inch, life's a cinch. Yard by yard, it is hard. Mile by mile, it's a trial."

Do you spend a lot of time worrying about the future? Your ideas about what might happen may not be based on verified information. These theories may leave you vulnerable to exaggerating problems and setting off a negative feedback loop. Your decisions based on inflated worries about the future may not be the most constructive. Perhaps you underestimate the possibility of change without knowing all the facts. Some may assume they are fortunetellers and decide:

This is how it is meant to be. There is no point trying.

I shouldn't bother with screening. They will just find something.

I won't be able to manage the finances or paperwork required.

I just know the odds are against me. There is no point in fighting.

When you focus on what is happening right now, you are less likely to get caught up in unproductive thoughts of what happened in the past that can't be changed or worries about what could happen in the future. What's more, when you keep your attention on the present, you are less likely to miss the preciousness of life at this moment.

Unproven Assumptions or Judgments

The last part of the definition of mindfulness is noticing reality without adding in unproven ideas or judgments. Let's take a closer look at judgments to illustrate the potential damage of these unconfirmed beliefs.

Judgments are emotionally charged personal opinions *added* to the facts. These assumptions assess the value or worth of a situation, person, or emotion as "good/bad" or "better/worse," or communicate what "should" be. They can be expressed in thoughts, in attitude, by the body, or in actions.

We make these judgments all the time. Can you recall a recent time you evaluated someone or something as "good/bad" or "better/worse"? I sure can! We often use these labels to try to specify consequences. I just told myself the last paragraph I wrote was "bad." My self-judgment was a way of expressing my view that I had not communicated effectively. The problem with taking my personal opinion as verified fact is compounded when I accept my own view as the definitive truth about my writing or self-worth.

Are you making judgments about the fact that you have cancer?

This should not be happening to me.

I shouldn't have cancer.

Cancer is unfair!

I should have had more healthy habits.

This is my fault.

Of course you want to be healthy! The wish for your reality to be different is understandable and is not a judgment. It does not change the fact that you have cancer. The **judgment comes when you add the *should* to that undesirable fact.**

Judgments that are ruled by extremes of emotion or logic don't provide a balanced or full picture of the situation. They can be confused with proven reality. Assumptions about how life "should be" intensify your emotions. You may be making decisions based on your wish to be in a situation that is more fair or tolerable than the actual situation. You can easily take your personal outlooks based on unreliable data as *the* definitive fact instead of a single momentary emotional reaction to the full situation. Effective choices require trustworthy, accurate information. **Judgments cloud the difference between reliable information and unproved ideas, making it harder to realistically see what is actually happening.**

Benefits of Mindfulness

You might be tempted to dismiss mindfulness as a current fad or decide these strategies will never work for you. Yet it may be worth your consideration as **research has shown that being aware of physical and emotional distress improves your ability to cope in many ways.** Mindfulness practice has been shown to help cancer patients:

- Lessen depression
- Decrease anxiety and stress
- Minimize difficulties with sleep and fatigue
- Improve quality of life

At a time when you may feel your ability to take charge of your body or how your life is going is limited, mindfulness may also be empowering as it has been proven to:

- Reduce ruminating thoughts
- Improve tolerance of physical pain
- Impact immune functioning
- Increase empathy/compassion

Last but not least, **paying attention to your body can be an important way to be more responsive to your health needs.** One man shared the way learning to pay attention to his body helped him to be clearer about whether he wanted or needed more or less water, food, caffeine, or pain meds. His experience may have been useful for a woman who ended up hospitalized for dehydration and a collapsed lung after disregarding her symptoms.

Mindfulness Skills

Let's look at how to use these skills. When you're mindful, you choose to try being **aware of what is happening at this moment.** You can get the fullest view of your circumstances by **observing and describing both your internal and external experience.** Your internal experience includes your feelings, thoughts, and sensations. Your external experience refers to the sights, sounds, smells, and tactile impressions in the world around you. The observations are most accurate when you **notice and label what you observe through your senses without adding unproven assumptions or judgments.**

Rest assured you do not need to be a monk, meditate, or even necessarily sit quietly for a period of time to be mindful. DBT mindfulness skills translate Eastern meditation practices into everyday life. You get some of the benefits of the traditional practices by noticing that your mind has inevitably wandered from what is happening right now and then bringing your attention back to the present.

Physical Sensations

Paying attention to your experience may be very new for you. See if you can take a moment right now to be curious and observe anything inside or around you that you hadn't been aware of until you stopped to look. Try to pause and see if you can notice at least two physical sensations.

Take a deep breath and slowly exhale. If it works for you, do your best to attempt to scan your body for any sense of tightness, ease, coolness, or warmth. Are you able to notice your heart rate? Initially, you may not recognize any sensations. Your head, throat, hands, and belly are good places to look. Perhaps you can feel your feet on the ground or the sensation of your body as it touches the chair. Maybe you can detect some tension in your muscles or pick up on the rise and fall of your chest as you breathe? This may all be too new, yet see if it's possible to be aware of sensations changing from one moment to the next. Can you detect them getting stronger, weaker, more or less vivid or intense?

Note: Your own wise mind is always the best guide about whether any suggestion in this book is useful for you. Feel free to stop if you find you become too agitated by noticing pain or other sensations.

Thoughts

Now try to observe your thoughts. Do your best to notice and identify the first two ideas that come to mind. **Observing thoughts is different from purposely thinking something.** The goal is to attempt to control your attention, not what you see. It may be difficult, but see if it's possible to watch your thoughts come and let them pass without holding on to them, as if they are going by on a conveyor belt.

Have you added any assumptions, judgments, explanations, or opinions? Don't criticize yourself for making judgments. We are often quick to decide there is something wrong with a natural reaction and judge ourselves for judging! Indeed, we make judgments all the time, including about this exercise or the way we do it. Being aware of how frequently we make them is the first step to minimizing them.

Emotions

Now see if it's possible to observe any emotions you're feeling. Are you worried, calm, annoyed, anxious, sad, irritable, frustrated, or angry? Perhaps you notice where in your body you feel the emotion and what it feels like. Recognizing and naming emotions is likely a new experience and not easy. Do as much as you can here and let that be good enough. You're still learning! In later chapters we present thoughts and physical responses common to particular emotions that may make identification easier.

Next let's put together what we've discussed to see how to use mindfulness to make effective decisions:

Steps for Effective Choices

- Name the decision.
- Observe and describe:
  - Sensations
  - Emotions
  - Thoughts
- Identify state of mind: emotion, reasonable, or wise.
- Take a balanced wise mind perspective.
  - Use accurate and reliable information.
    - Minimize added judgments.
    - Focus on the present.
  - Broaden perspective for more complete story.
    - Challenge black-or-white notions.
    - Consider additional points of view.
    - Balance facts *and* your preferences/values.

As an example, let's follow the way Sara uses these steps to make a decision about having a mastectomy. She begins by trying to be open to her current experience without pushing away or holding on to feelings, thoughts, or sensations that are particularly comfortable or unpleasant. She attempts to let her impressions come up and then pass by like the constant waves of the ocean. Easier said than done!

She does her best to notice her **bodily sensations** by observing and labeling information from eyes, ears, nose, skin, and tongue. She recognizes and acknowledges:

I have a lump in my throat.

I am looking down at the floor.

My hands are clammy.

My heart is racing.

I have butterflies in my stomach.

I feel unsteady on my feet.

Next she tries to be aware of her **thoughts:**

I don't need to do this surgery.

Can I really die if I don't do this? I have so much I still want to do with my life!

I don't want to feel deformed.

Are there surgical options that will make a difference?

I shouldn't have to sacrifice the sensation of a natural breast.

Is there really a choice to consider if my life is at risk?

I want a second opinion.

I am too overwhelmed to make this decision. I can't even keep track of what they are telling me or remember my questions.

Will I be less of a woman?

Will my husband still find me attractive?

If I do this surgery, I want to wake up and feel intact.

Her goal is to stand back and notice these thoughts without getting caught up in their content. She tries to **describe** her thinking:

A wish to question and reject facts appears.

Judgments crop up about needing surgery or how I might look.

Doubt and questions come up.

Self-critical ideas occur to me.

Ideas appear about how my husband or I will feel about me in the future.

Notions change rapidly and can reappear.

Personal preferences come up.

When she observes and describes her **emotions,** she recognizes:

Fear

Anxiety

Anger

Agitation

Apprehension

Sadness

Worry

When Sara is able to pay careful attention to her feelings and thoughts, she sees how swiftly her emotions and ideas continually shift and then recur, like the constant motion of the seesaw.

Next she realizes that she is in emotion mind, recognizing that her thinking is strongly influenced by her fear and worry. If she were in reasonable mind, the statistics alone might dominate her thoughts without allowing consideration of any doubts, questions, or personal preferences. She hopes to avoid staying on one extreme *or* the other and to find a middle place that balances the facts *and* her feelings.

Her goal is to not overlook her capacity for wisdom and make her decision from a balanced wise mind. After noticing she is letting her emotions govern her thinking, Sara pauses to attempt to get the objective and subjective information in perspective. She wants to be sure her decision is based on accurate and reliable information, so she tries to pay attention only to what she observes through her senses. Her assumptions and judgments are ideas that are only in her head and therefore cannot be observed. She tries to be aware of all her *should*s as well as her ideas about certain feelings or circumstances being good or bad/better or worse. Sara tries to let go of these judgments. She makes an effort to be aware of when she is getting ahead of herself with many worries about what might happen in the future and tries to stay focused on current facts she knows for sure.

Sara also wonders how else she might respond effectively. Can she expand from a narrow outlook and challenge some of her black-or-white notions? Her goal is to broaden her perspective to get a fuller view. She attempts to zoom out as if she is looking at her situation from a helicopter above to consider additional points of view or interpretations. She recognizes that she doesn't have to be totally overwhelmed *or* in full control. Perhaps there is a middle ground. She considers asking for help and draws up a list of her questions and concerns in advance of her next appointment. She decides to have someone go with her to write down everything the doctor says.

While Sara might not be able to have all of her wishes, her wise mind considers whether it is possible to balance the medical facts and her preferences. Perhaps she does have to accept that this is a surgery that is recommended for her health. Is there a chance that she does not have to give up everything that is important to her? She decides to inquire whether there are medical options appropriate for her that can address any of her concerns and preferences.

Practice Exercises

Honing mindfulness skills may help to ensure that your decisions are based on the most reliable and complete information. These skills help balance emotion and reasonable mind to ensure a fuller, more accurate view of the situation. Like any new ability, the skills of observing, describing, minimizing judgments, and taking a wise mind perspective require practice. Do your best to try to use them when you can without judging yourself over skills that take time to master. Below are some ways that can be used to sharpen your skills.

Practicing Paying Full Attention to Experience by Observing and Describing

It may be easier to begin to work on these mindfulness skills with an experience that is less emotionally charged than something related to cancer. A good first exercise to consider trying is to **observe your bodily**

sensations as you walk. Try to find a place where you are not likely to be disturbed. See if you can:

- Bring a childlike wonder or curiosity to your experience as if you are walking for the first time.
- Feel the air as it touches your face, hands, and any other exposed areas.
- Listen to the sounds around you.
- Notice your breath at either your belly or the tip of your nose as it comes in and goes out.
- Walk slowly.
- Try to pay attention to the sensations of your feet on the ground as you walk, while resisting the temptation to put words, explanations, or evaluations to the experience:
  - Move one foot forward and see if you can detect the sensations of lifting in your foot, leg, and the rest of your body.
  - Pay attention as you place your foot on the ground in front of you. Are you aware of feeling the heel of your foot? Can you discern the sensation of each of your toes on the ground or bottom of your shoe?
  - Next purposefully lift and move the other foot forward and notice all the sensations involved in placing it back on the ground.
- Notice the thoughts that arise:
  - See if you can discern judgments. Do you have ideas about the worth of this exercise? Are you rating yourself on how well you think you're doing?
  - Attempt to be aware of the notions but not get caught up in them.
  - Try to let thoughts come and pass by like something moving on a conveyor belt or leaves floating down a river.
  - When your mind inevitably wanders, give an understanding smile as you realize you're learning. You're practicing a new skill. Return your attention to the sensations of walking at this moment. You're beginning to train your mind!

Next, try to **describe your experience.** Here you want to name the body sensations, emotions, and thoughts that you are aware of while practicing. The ideal is to put your experience into words, labeling *only* what you observe at this moment without adding judgments, assumptions, premature conclusions, or other theories. Some people find writing down the description to be a very useful practice.

A sample of describing the walking exercise might be:

- I felt the gentle breeze on my face.
- I heard a whirring sound.
- I felt my breath at the tip of my nostrils as I inhaled.
- I noticed the heel of my foot. I was aware of the sensation in my big toe as it touched my shoe.
- I questioned whether this exercise was stupid.
- Annoyance came up.
- I was not aware of any sensations as I lifted my leg.
- Self-consciousness arose.
- Judgments came to mind. I told myself that I was no good at this. I questioned whether this stuff could be helpful.
- I realized I hadn't been thinking about my cancer for these few minutes.
- Evaluating thoughts arose. I decided this exercise might be helpful.
- Remorse came up.
- I realized that I first assumed the whirring sound was a lawn mower in the distance. The sound could have been another garden tool, power tool, or something else I haven't imagined.
- I thought I should really be getting back to work.
- I noticed my mind had drifted from paying attention to walking.
- I began to pay attention to my walking again.
- Pride arose.

Practicing Wise Mind

Finding wise mind consistently takes a lot of practice. Below are some ideas for practice.

Stone on the Lake

Imagine that you are by a clear blue lake on a beautiful sunny day. Then picture yourself as a small flake of stone, flat and light. Imagine that you have been tossed out onto the lake and are now gently, slowly floating through the calm, clear blue water to the lake's smooth sand bottom.

- Notice what you see, what you feel as you float down, perhaps in slow circles, floating toward the bottom. As you reach the bottom of the lake, settle your attention there within yourself.
- Try to pay attention to the serenity of the lake; become aware of the calmness and quiet deep within.
- As you reach the center of yourself, settle your attention there.

Walking Down the Spiral Stairs

Imagine that within you is a spiral staircase, winding down to your very center. Starting at the top, walk very slowly down the staircase, going deeper and deeper within yourself.

- Notice the sensations. Rest by sitting on a step or turn on lights on the way down if you wish. Do not force yourself farther than you want to go. Notice the quiet. As you reach the center of yourself, settle your attention there—perhaps in your gut or abdomen.

Dropping into the Pauses between Inhaling and Exhaling

- Breathing in, notice the pause after inhaling (top of breath).
- Breathing out, notice the pause after exhaling (bottom of breath).
- At each pause, let yourself "fall into" the center space within the pause.

Practicing Being Nonjudgmental

- Describe *only* the facts that you observe with your senses without evaluations, assumptions, or comparisons.

- Try to notice how things are without adding "should," "good or bad," "better or worse."

- Pay attention to and try to change any judgmental facial expressions, postures, or voice tones (even the ones in your head!).

- Notice the inevitable judgments that come up without giving yourself a hard time. Consider gently saying, "A judgment occurred to me."

- To become more aware of how often you become judgmental you might consider counting judgmental thoughts and statements by manually clicking a counter or marking on a piece of paper.

- Noticing judgments is an ongoing process for us all.

Next we turn to understanding and managing emotions.

THREE

How to Manage Strong Emotions

Have you ever had any of these thoughts?

I feel like I'm being hit by a tidal wave of emotions.

Am I just going to break down?

Should I just try to ignore these painful feelings?

I better keep these intense emotions to myself.

I don't want anyone to think I'm weak and pity me.

Intense feelings can be difficult to handle at any time. The challenges can seem even harder when you're living with cancer. So many new and unpredictable things are happening in your body. If you also feel as if powerful emotions are threatening to overwhelm your mind, you may feel even more vulnerable.

When I had cancer, I actually worried about being out of control and had an intense dream.

I was driving an unreliable car in the pouring rain. I was in unfamiliar territory. The place on the dashboard where the GPS should be was an empty dark hole. I tried unsuccessfully to get to the maps on my phone. I couldn't get through when I tried to make a phone call for assistance. I thought I should just pull over but couldn't stop. The rain became blinding, and I was in a flooded area, engulfed by water. I was unable to control what was happening. The car was sinking with me inside!

I woke myself up yelling, "Help, help!" The powerful dread, pounding heart, sickness in my stomach, and tightness in my chest remained for some time after I was awake.

Whether you have cancer or not, no one likes to be worried, sad, or irritable. Yet these feelings can be common reactions to life with cancer. Even knowing that others may feel as we do, we can give ourselves a hard time about having intense emotions. Do you tell yourself you should be handling your feelings differently? Are you looking for ways to manage strong emotions? How can you do that?

DBT teaches that although you can't change unpredictable and uncontrollable situations, **you can change *how* you respond.** You can regain a sense of control and emotional balance by learning how to regulate strong emotions. In this chapter we offer ways to constructively accept feelings without being consumed by them. We explain how emotions function and present concrete skills to manage powerful feelings, as well as strategies to calm yourself in the moment.

Understanding Emotions

Emotions have a bad reputation. We make judgments about strong feelings. We may decide some emotions are good ones *or* bad ones. We may believe we should avoid certain feelings *or* they may overwhelm us. The fact is that suppressing emotions can get in the way of effective coping. Blocking feelings intensifies them. Studies report that cancer patients who could understand, categorize, and label their emotions showed improved emotional coping and other health benefits such as lower levels of inflammation. We are going to show you how to do this.

To get a fuller understanding of emotions, let's start by looking at their positive aspects. Surprisingly, they can be very helpful.

Emotions Can Be Constructive Guides to Action

They can **give you messages about the safety of a situation,** letting you know whether or not you need to be alert and aware of danger. They can also **motivate you to overcome obstacles and take productive action.**

- **Fear** can communicate the need to escape from danger, to run from a lion or immediately consult a doctor.

- **Anger** can mobilize you to protect yourself against a physical or emotional threat, to play harder on the football field, or speak up when you are not getting the help you need.

- **Anxiety** can be a sign that you need to respond to and act on your worry, to study for that test or call the doctor.

- **Sadness** tells you that it might be useful to reach out to others for support.

Emotions Provide Quick, Nonverbal Communication

Your facial expression, body language, and tone of voice can intentionally or unintentionally send messages to people around you. Expressions of empathy and compassion have been called the **language of connection.** Indeed, openly showing feeling has been found to communicate trustworthiness and increase social connection.

So how do feelings stir up an unhelpful reaction?

Negative Feedback Loop:
An Unproductive Cycle of Emotions

Let's assume Sara is anxiously awaiting an overdue call from her doctor with information vital to her course of treatment. Many of us would feel agitated in this situation. Sara's initial response, frustration, is called the **primary emotion.** Physiologically this emotion, or any emotion for that matter, lasts only for approximately 90 seconds.

After that minute and a half, we have additional reactions, presumptions, and judgments about the situation. For example, Sara might now think:

This is outrageous!

Does my doctor know what it is like to be waiting?

I am so aggravated. She is unreliable.

How am I going to trust someone so insensitive?

The doctor must be waiting for more time to talk because the news is so bad.

Am I just a bitchy, demanding patient?

These opinions and doubts can stir up **secondary emotions** such as indignation, mistrust, anger, apprehension, anxiety, or shame. Sara's initial reaction of frustration is now maintained and/or intensified by these thoughts, body sensations, and emotional reactions that impact each other. Her subsequent feelings may be based on judgments about her frustration, as well as thoughts about the way her feelings can impact her and her relationships. These secondary emotions are also referred to as the second arrow because she is "hit" again!

Marsha uses the expression **"emotions love themselves"** to describe the way experiencing an emotion can leave you even more sensitive to other information that confirms or magnifies that feeling. You can feel flooded by these secondary feelings and unable to find the off switch, like when the gas pedal in a car is stuck to the floor.

Sara's initial frustration may have been useful if it rallied her to check with her doctor, yet now she may be **holding on to feelings past their usefulness.** If Sara focuses on ideas that confirm her feelings, the frustration and indignation may intensify. Now she is angry. Physical expressions of anger, such as a flushed face and feeling on the verge of tears, may now unwittingly reinforce her emotion. She may make judgments about her doctor that may or may not be accurate. Suppose she begins to worry that her care may not be reliable. She may then become critical and judgmental of herself for feeling so agitated, possibly stirring up shame. She is likely already anxious about the news. Now this flood of secondary ongoing emotions not clearly based on facts can get in the way of her effective coping.

So let's look at how can you reduce this unproductive cycling of emotions.

How to Regulate an Emotion

- Allow yourself to be aware of how you are feeling.
- Pause to observe your emotional experience.

- Pay attention to where and how the feeling is expressed in your body.
  - Notice your thoughts.
- Describe the experience.
  - Name the emotion you wish to control.
  - Label the prompting event.
  - Identify physical reactions and judgments/assumptions about the event.
- Check the facts.
  - Are your ideas verified by facts?
  - Are you assuming a threat? If so, name it and assess the likelihood of its happening.
- Ask wise mind.
  - Does the emotion or its intensity fit the facts?
  - Consider other possible perspectives.
  - Decide whether it is in your interest to express or act on the emotion.

Facing Feelings

The first step of emotion regulation is to pause **to allow your feelings.** We can't control an emotion we don't acknowledge. We are trying to manage feelings, not block them! In fact, **complete emotional control is neither possible nor desirable.** Trying to avoid emotions can be like playing with one of those Chinese paper finger traps. The more you try to pull away, the more you get stuck. Recall that blocking feelings actually intensifies them. What's more, when we don't acknowledge our emotions, we can miss their useful message.

Why do we try to avoid feelings? At times we may believe the myth that accepting the emotion means approving of or consenting to feeling as we do. We may also worry that admitting a feeling will open the floodgates and overwhelm us with uncontrollable emotion.

When I was anticipating surgery, I imagined that if I allowed any anxiety or sadness to surface I was giving in to those feelings. Like many people, I made judgments about my emotions. I was concerned that I would pay a price for showing "negative, unacceptable" emotions. I thought I *should* be more positive and was critical of myself for feeling apprehensive or gloomy. I worried that any fear or anguish might define me as weak or selfish. I covered my feelings to protect my self-image and avoid shame or pity. I wanted to ensure I didn't appear vulnerable to myself or to anyone else.

The goal of emotion regulation is to find a balanced place between avoiding feelings and allowing them without being overwhelmed by them. The ideal is to accept emotions, not push them away, hold on to them, or amplify them. I love an image a wise Zen teacher shared with me. He told me to think about lightly holding my feelings in a flat open palm instead of using a tight fist to try to hold on to them or punch them away. With an open palm we try to **allow the feeling to come and then let it go,** like surfing rising and falling waves.

I saw firsthand that trying to block emotions does not work. As much as I tried to avoid any anxiety or sadness, my feelings showed up anyway. My sister had offered to be at the hospital, and I said it wasn't necessary. On the morning of my surgery, I was surprised by my strong desire to connect to the family of my childhood and now wanted my sister with me. With the reality of the surgery staring me in the face, I then asked her to make the long trip to the hospital. At the time, I neither understood my emotional reaction nor was aware of what I was feeling. Yet luckily I respected their message to reach out for support. Blessedly, so did my sister. She came.

I nearly missed a valuable message from feelings I judged as destructive and did not want to accept. I was so busy trying to be strong that I was not able to ask people to support me or allow them in to do so. I later learned that my emotions did not have to be on or off. I could cope more effectively by allowing my feelings *and* learning to regulate their intensity. I could learn how to acknowledge a constructive message from my feelings *and* control emotions when they escalated and/or persisted unproductively.

Now let's follow the way Sara might manage her anger about not hearing from her doctor in the expected time frame as an example of how to regulate emotion.

Pause to Observe the Emotional Experience

Paying attention to where and how the emotion is expressed can help Sara recognize the factors in the feedback loop. She begins by stopping to recognize how she is feeling. Unlike me, Sara is in emotion mind and allows her feelings. She acknowledges her intense irritation. She attempts to pay attention to her thoughts without automatically accepting everything that comes to mind as fact. She makes an effort to notice where in her body she is reacting, discerning her flushed face, the tension in her jaw, and her clenched hands.

Describe the Experience

Sara tries to put words to a full picture of her inner experience. Labeling reactions is a crucial step in emotion regulation as it can help identify cues that may be intensifying the emotion by triggering a negative feedback loop. What's more, identifying a feeling literally helps to decrease its intensity.

Name the Emotion You Are Trying to Control

"Name it to tame it" reflects the research showing that **labeling an emotion calms the central nervous system.** Also recall that cancer patients who could categorize and label their emotions showed improved coping as well as other health benefits. Sara identifies her anger.

Naming your feelings is not always easy. I learned that it is even harder to label emotions that we are trying to avoid. At times we just don't know what we are feeling or how our emotions connect to our actions. Our secondary emotions can make it even harder to recognize a primary emotion. In the following chapters we offer additional ways to help you recognize the most common emotions that occur with cancer.

Label the Prompting Event

The next step for Sara in describing her experience is to try to recognize the source of her feeling. It is not always easy to identify what instigates an

emotion. We typically think of the prompting event as an external experience, such as her not hearing from the doctor as needed and expected.
Yet Sara's anger may also be triggered by an internal experience such as
a physical sensation like pain. It is also possible that ruminating thoughts
such as fear about the news and/or her indignation refueling itself may be
perpetuating her anger.

Identify Physical Reactions and Judgments/Assumptions

Now Sara tries to label her judgments or assumptions and put words to
the way her body is responding. Identifying her reactions may help her be
more aware of cues that may be intensifying her emotion.

She notices that her body expresses anger in her flushed face, the
tension in her jaw, and her clenched hands. She recognizes that she is
making black-or-white judgments about her doctor and herself. She
labels her assumptions that either her doctor is insensitive, unreliable,
and untrustworthy *or* she is just too demanding. Sara sees that she is also
imagining that the news is bad.

Check the Facts

When the outcome is very important and/or the threat is likely to become
reality, we are even more apt to have an intense and enduring reaction.
Sara's anger makes sense if she has repeatedly had unresponsive medical
care and feels her health or peace of mind is compromised.

Yet it's very valuable for Sara to be sure her assumptions are correct.
Have her ideas been confirmed by facts? Although there may be a possibility her worst nightmares are true, her worries may not always be justified or give a complete picture of the situation. Believing inaccurate ideas
can make her more emotional than may be warranted. She doesn't want
to add unnecessary distress by incorrectly assuming bad news.

Her goal is to check out the accuracy of her assumptions, including
why she hasn't heard from her doctor. She tries to name any threats she
imagines. She recognizes that the threats are the possibility of getting
unwelcome news, the risk of receiving insensitive, unreliable care, or the
possibility that she is a difficult patient.

Wise Mind

The next step is for Sara to use wise mind to take a wider, more balanced perspective. Are there other ways to look at her situation to get a fuller picture about her doctor and herself? Does the intensity of her anger fit the facts of her circumstances? She considers:

> *Are there other reasons the doctor may not have called? Could there be an administrative problem at her office? Could I have missed the call?*
>
> *Is it possible that getting back to me is one of many priorities and she is caught up with other patients? When I stop to think about it, is my doctor usually reliable?*
>
> *Is my irritation stronger than the facts warrant? Could my agitation be stronger because I'm awaiting important news about my health?*
>
> *I am indignant right now. Yet I am not usually an angry, demanding patient. Does my anger really define me?*

Deciding Whether to Express Feelings

There is a difference between a natural urge to act on emotions and actually expressing them at this moment. You have a choice. Your wise mind can be a valuable guide to help you consider whether it is in your interest to act on your feelings right now.

When feelings are not confirmed by fact, the most constructive decision is often *not* to act right away. Sara's experience with her doctor is that she *is* normally reliable. She recognizes that her feelings are stronger than the facts warrant and decides it is not in her interest to express her feelings to the doctor at this time. She does not want to risk compromising a relationship with someone she needs to rely on. Instead Sara decides to pause, correct her assumptions, and try to regulate her emotions.

On the other hand, what can Sara do if her assumptions are accurate? Suppose Sara's doctor is not as responsive as she wants and needs. She may still wisely decide to try to reduce the intensity of her anger. Yet now it may be in her interest to address the problem by expressing her feelings and taking action.

Problem Solving to Take Action

Let's look at problem-solving strategies to use when assumptions do fit the facts.

- Describe the problem.
- Check the facts.
- Identify the goal.
- Brainstorm lots of solutions.
- Choose a solution that fits the goal and is likely to work.
- Act.

The problem is Sara's worry that her doctor is not as responsive as she wants or needs. In this case, when she checks her facts, her assumptions are correct, and her indignation is understandable. Her goal is to have a good working relationship with a medical provider who is responsive and provides good medical care.

At this point she thinks through possible actions. For example, she can acknowledge her disappointment to herself. She can share her feelings with a loved one. She can talk to someone in her doctor's office. She can speak directly to her doctor. Or she can change doctors.

If Sara decides to talk directly to her doctor, she will want to know how to express herself while protecting a relationship with someone she needs to rely on. Chapter 8 covers strategies for communication with medical providers and offers interpersonal skills Sara can use to talk effectively with her doctor.

Short-Term Ways to Tolerate Intense Distress

At times pain may be extreme. What can you do if your feelings seem too intense (over 80 on a scale of 1–100) to face at this moment? Your immediate priority may be to get enough relief to hold it together. Perhaps you feel too overwhelmed to think through all the steps of emotion regulation. These strategies to tolerate distress do not solve the problem, yet they do offer ways to get through a difficult time by changing the physical input to the feedback loop.

Paced Breathing

Paced breathing is an effective way to promote calm feelings by slowing your heart rate. Even better, the skill can be used in public without others knowing. For example, Sara can use this skill if her anger remains too intense or persistent, yet she has to sit in her doctor's office and wait for test results.

Calm is promoted by taking a longer exhale than inhale. When you change your body chemistry by altering your breathing pattern, you cut off the physical input to a negative loop of danger. Slowing down the heart rate activates the parasympathetic nervous system. **If you have any breathing issues, consult your doctor before using this skill.**

To use paced breathing:

- Slow down your pace of breathing to an average of five or six breaths per minute.
- Try to breathe deeply from your abdomen.
- Inhale to a slow count of 4.
- Pause.
- Try to exhale to a count of 6 or if possible to 8. Repeat.

Paired Muscle Relaxation

This strategy ties muscle relaxation to exhalation to reduce physical tension and promote calm. As with every suggestion in this book, use your wise mind to be sure the following practice is helpful to you.

The steps to take are:

- Inhale as you stiffen and tighten your muscles, but not so much as to cause a cramp.
- Pay attention to the tension in your body for 4–5 seconds.

- Exhale for 6–7 seconds while softening the tension. Say the word *relax* in your mind as you slump like a rag doll.
- Bring your attention to your **facial muscles.**
  - Wrinkle your forehead and then let go.
  - Squeeze your eyes tightly and then relax them.
  - Furrow your brows and then soften.
  - Scrunch your cheeks and nose tightly and then release.
  - Grind your teeth and then let your whole mouth and jaw be slack with tongue relaxed and your teeth slightly apart.
  - Tightly pucker your lips and then let the corners of your lips relax and turn up slightly with a half smile and calm facial expression.
- Notice your **shoulders, arms, and hands.**
  - As you take a deep breath, bring your tightened fists up to your ears and shrug your shoulders.
  - As you let out the breath, drop your arms down and turn your unclenched hands outward with your palms up and your fingers relaxed.
- Focus on your **torso, legs, and feet.**
  - Hold your stomach in tightly and squeeze your buttocks together. Then soften.
  - Tense your thighs and calves and then release.
  - Flex your ankles, curl your toes, and then let them slacken.

Some find that even briefly bringing their attention to any area of physical discomfort is too agitating. If sensations are too overwhelming, shift to another part of the body, avoid that area, or do not use this practice.

The more often you do this technique, the more effective it becomes at helping to promote calm. The first time you try it you want to be in a quiet place and have plenty of time. As you improve, attempt to use it in many different settings so it becomes possible to use this strategy wherever you are and whenever you need it.

The next three chapters demonstrate how to apply this emotion regulation framework to the most common emotions in dealing with cancer. As it is sometimes difficult to know and identify feelings, we include specific ways to help you recognize and label fear, sadness, and anger. We also offer more short-term ways to tolerate distress.

FOUR

Managing Fear, Anxiety, and Stress

People react to cancer in different ways. Over 51% of cancer patients surveyed said their most important need was to cope with fear. Although fear and anxiety may provide valuable information about a threat of danger, these understandable feelings are often distressing and upsetting. Are you assuming frightening things are going to happen? Are you afraid you will lose capacities, relationships, dignity, or even your life? Do you believe constant worry protects you by keeping you vigilant to potential dangers? Perhaps you're concerned that your fear or anxiety is too intense and destructive. Have these emotions gotten in the way of doing what you need to do to take good care of yourself? Have you added the impact of stress to a long list of concerns?

It's possible to find a fitting place for understandable reactions to cancer. This chapter offers ways to find a wise mind balanced response to the inevitable stress of living with this disease. We introduce the coping strategies of opposite action, self-talk, and cope ahead to reduce fear and anxiety that may be more extreme than is in your interest. In addition, we suggest more ways to tolerate distress in the short term.

Negative Feedback Loop of Fear, Anxiety, and Stress

Let's take a look at a framework for understanding the fear, anxiety, and stress that can be an inherent part of dealing with cancer. In a frightening situation like cancer, fear often makes sense. Recall that fear mobilizes a physiological stress response to prepare you to take protective action from an immediate danger. The body works together with thoughts to avoid harm. After the danger passes, the body's stress response usually resets to normal and frightening thoughts subside.

Yet for many people cancer also highlights the reality of living with an uncertain future. At times it may be unclear whether there is an ongoing threat, and anxiety or apprehension about what *might* happen is understandable. The trouble may come when anxiety's ongoing nervous thoughts and the same stressful body reaction as fear set off a vicious cycle. The more anxious you are, the more distressed you may become. The more distressed you feel, the more things you may worry about. The more frightened and anxious you feel, the more stressed your body remains.

Mindfully pausing to pay attention to all the parts of your experience may help you be clearer about where you may be able to make changes to break off this unproductive cycle.

Facing Fear, Anxiety, and Stress

Recall the first step is to pause to acknowledge how you feel. Not so easy to do here. The problem can be that when we are afraid, many of us are inclined to run in the other direction—physically and emotionally. Some of us do anything we can to get away from that raw panicked feeling. I even avoid scary movies because I don't like to feel ill at ease and on the edge of my seat.

Judgments about fear and anxiety or assumptions about what the emotions say about us can keep us from allowing these feelings. One man told me he believed his fear was a weakness. He falsely believed the myth that acknowledging fear and anxiety is the same as passively accepting cancer, giving up without fighting for his health, or believing that he can't manage those feelings. Another woman said she didn't want to even use the word *fear* in relation to her cancer. She regarded the word as taboo because she did not want fear to rule her life.

Are we now suggesting that you need to allow yourself to be aware of feeling frightened to be able to reduce your fear? As contradictory as it may sound, recall that accepting your feelings, acknowledging that you're afraid, is an essential step to both protect yourself and cope with how scared you can feel.

In fact, acknowledging fear helps you protect and defend yourself or people you care about. Noticing your fear ensures you don't miss a signal to brace for danger and act on the threat. Allowing realistic fear can motivate you to take difficult action—to run into that burning building to save your child!

Looking fear in the eye and facing threats can also help you make effective decisions. The same woman who did not want to use the word *fear* also said she was aware that her worry about her health had mobilized her to make healthier choices about how she lived. After she bravely looked at her risk of recurrence, she changed her diet and started exercising regularly.

You are at greater risk of being ruled by panic when you deny the feeling. Facing the ongoing fear that contributes to anxiety can help minimize its power over you. Pausing to allow yourself to pay attention to your fearful thoughts and feelings may help you notice that they can come and go. It's possible that the process can also help you separate yourself from what you observe and take your fear less personally. You may see that your fear is not a statement about you that has to rule your life. As a result, you also may start to be less judgmental of yourself and actually feel less afraid.

In the same way, it's very important to accept that stress is an unavoidable part of all of our lives. Cancer or no cancer, stress is a natural response to life's inevitable challenges and the need to tolerate uncertainty. Of course you're stressed by cancer. Recognizing that your stress is not your fault may help you be less self-critical. You may actually feel less anxious or stressed.

Recognizing the Emotion

To control fear, try your best to allow yourself to be aware of and acknowledge your feelings by paying attention to where and how the emotion is communicated. Some people have no trouble noticing their fear and anxiety. They know all too well how they're feeling. Consider Keisha, who is hyperalert to her aches and pains, worrying that every physical sensation implies a negative prognosis. Her apprehension about bad news leaves her nauseous. She dreads doctor's appointments, which she finds terrifying, and fantasizes about just staying home. Yet like me, others may put so much energy into avoiding their emotion that they find it difficult to recognize how they feel.

To help you identify your feelings, let's look at some of the common ways fear may be expressed in your mind, body, and thoughts.

"Name It to Tame It"

Remember that labeling the experience helps to quiet the feeling. Knowing many ways to identify and name an emotion can help you to both recognize what you may be feeling and calm yourself.

Some of the most common words used to describe fear include:

Anxiety	Hysteria	Tenseness
Apprehension	Jumpiness	Terror
Dread	Nervousness	Uneasiness
Edginess	Overwhelm	Worry
Fright	Panic	
Horror	Shock	

It can also be useful to notice and label that you're experiencing stress. See if you can take a step back to identify that you feel stressed without adding a negative judgment about health implications or your ability to cope. Indeed, taking this step gives you more reason to feel confident about your coping, as mindfulness strategies have been shown to build more resilience to stress.

Physical Expression of Fear and Anxiety

Physical sensations should always be reviewed with your doctor. In addition, it may be useful for you, like Keisha, to have a sense of what physical reactions may also be expressions of fear and anxiety. Let's look at where and how fear can commonly be communicated in the face and body.

Are you aware of whether your teeth are clenched or if there is a scowl on your face? Are you crying? Eyes wide open? Mouth slack? Are you sweating? Shivering? Do you discern a lump in your throat? How about butterflies in your stomach or trembling limbs? Pressure, tightness, aches, or heat in your head, throat, chest, and/or belly may be signs of fear and anxiety. Your doctor can verify the possibility that breathlessness and/or a fast heartbeat may be emotionally driven.

Your tense posture may also be a clue to the presence of fear. Do you feel like a bundle of tight muscles defending your existence? Is your head forward? Are your shoulders knotted or hunched forward? Have you crossed your arms? Is your back hunched or your chest sunken? When I stopped to scan my body, I noticed the rigid, tight way I was holding my arms and hands. I was a lot tenser than I realized.

When a fear response gets locked into your nervous system, the tension in your mind and body may perpetuate the emotional reaction beyond the initial physiological 90 seconds. Ongoing fear may also impact digestion with diarrhea, constipation, vomiting, or an increase or decrease in appetite. Again as with any symptom, be sure to consult your doctor.

Physical sensations can also retrigger painful emotions. One person realized that she became panicked when she smelled the same cleaning fluid that was used in the hospital during her stem cell transplant. The odor brought back painful sensory memories, and she felt flooded with anxiety. Another man realized that when he felt tired he was reminded of being unwell, and his fatigue triggered anxiety.

Thoughts That Express Fear and Anxiety

How might fear and anxiety show up in your thoughts? When we think we're in danger, we can narrow our attention to be hypervigilant to any risk. Fear and anxiety may be conveyed by incessant worried ideas about danger and assumptions of the worst outcome.

Keisha felt it was her job to scan for danger. Part of her believed her constant worry protected her and prepared her for a difficult future. When she noticed a cramp in her stomach, she assumed the new physical symptom meant her cancer had spread. She decided she should be resting more to conserve her energy and stopped taking the walks she loves.

Paying attention to whether you're staying in the present can be very useful in managing unproductive anxiety. Do you tell yourself stories about what could go wrong in the future and, like Keisha, anticipate new medical problems? Are you assuming your current problems will exist for the rest of your life? Do you find yourself imagining helplessness, suffering, or pain that doesn't exist right now?

See if you can also notice your judgments and assumptions. Are you, like many of us, self-critical about having many worries? Are you judging yourself for having unconstructive fear? Have you assumed your stress is a sign that you can't cope or your anxiety is making you worse? Are you ashamed of being so frightened? Keisha told herself that others didn't worry as much as she did. She decided she was letting fear and anxiety rule her life. She started calling herself "Nervous Nellie," invalidating her understandable concerns.

It's important for you, like Keisha, to keep in mind that fear and anxiety are understandable responses to cancer. Your judgments or well-meaning suggestions from others that you *should* "think positive" instead of being frightened, worried, or stressed can be invalidating. The message to deny or disregard negative feelings is unrealistic and may trivialize your pain and distress. What's more, a positive-thinking mantra can be an unfair burden if it implies that your natural feelings are simply the result of a bad attitude or if it leaves you blaming yourself for your medical status.

The most constructive way to deal with fearful and anxious thoughts is to notice them. Do your best to label that you are worrying without making judgments. Then attempt to let the thought go. Each time you identify an anxious thought you are mindfully training yourself not to stay with these concerns. While it may seem difficult, see if it's possible to imagine putting those thoughts on a conveyor belt and letting them pass by.

Check the Facts

When the cycle of anxiety gets started, we're vulnerable to fretful beliefs that may not have a rational basis. Try to check the facts to be sure your fear is realistic and there is actually as much danger as you imagine. Those anxious ideas may not be based in fact. You want to be sure that both your medical and emotional assumptions are accurate. Who needs added anxiety about fears unlikely to happen? Checking the facts gives you the opportunity to reset the stress response in your body by letting go of unrealistic concerns whenever possible.

Keisha assumes her medical provider is going to give her bad news. Is she correct? Cancer can run the spectrum from your ultimately being fine to the illness being life altering to your being likely to die. Are you as clear as you can be as to where your cancer stands? Are you giving up things that are important to you without being sure that is necessary? Keisha is assuming that the only explanation for her cramp is that her cancer has spread. She needs to assess the likelihood that her belief is accurate and that she really is advised to give up her beloved walks.

Wise Mind

There are times that fear makes sense but may not be useful. Ask your wise mind whether your emotion is more intense than is in your interest at this point. Have justifiable feelings become counterproductive, stirring up more anxiety? Is your constant anxiety providing more help or harm? Do you want to reduce the emotion?

After Keisha checked the facts with her doctor, she found that her cramp had no implications for her cancer or her treatment. Her PET scan showed no spread of her cancer. Both her medical assumptions and her beliefs were incorrect. Keisha saw that although her fear may have been understandable, she was adding unnecessary worries that intensified her problems. Her wise mind helped her take a more balanced perspective. She realized that her anxiety threatened to get in the way of her medical treatment and pursuing a beloved activity. She recognized that acting on her fear by avoiding the doctor or giving up her walks was not in her interest. At that point it was important that Keisha try not to give herself a hard time about her reaction. Many of us worry that things are worse than they actually turn out to be.

Opposite Action

There also may be times when intense fear is justified but still not in your interest. Opposite action for fear is based on effectively proven exposure-based treatments for anxiety disorders. It can help you cope when you need to change what you're doing or if the intensity of your fright is getting in the way of things you really need to do immediately. This strategy may help Keisha get herself to the doctor's office even if her fear is understandable yet unproductive.

The idea is to act totally opposite to the emotional urge that is common to the emotion. The most typical urge in response to fear is avoidance. When we're frightened, we may want to run away and hide from how we feel at that moment. We may look for any way possible to try to stop what we're feeling. Some of us go online, eat more, shop more, and/or use alcohol or drugs. Sometimes we lash out at others. We might feel desperate to distract ourselves from what we're feeling. The objective of opposite action is to go toward the thing you are afraid of, to approach instead of run away.

It can be hard to face frightening things, so you want to try to practice opposite action as fully as you can. The skill is most effective if you combine it with ways to use your body and thoughts to cue emotions that are the opposite of anxiety.

Physical Cues

Posture

Keisha might do her best to throw herself into going to the doctor by trying to use a confident tone and keep her head and eyes up. Her goal is to take an assertive body posture, holding her shoulders back and relaxed and standing up straight as she encourages herself to walk in.

Breath

Recall that paying attention to your breath can be a valuable way to refocus attention and calm the body by regulating a rapid heartbeat. Keisha may consider evenly pacing her breath to a 6-second inhale and 6-second exhale. Coherent breath can be effective to manage anxiety when you need to settle down enough to do something like get to the doctor. Dr. Richard Brown, author of *The Healing Power of Breath*, reports that coherent breath has been shown to help every system in the body and brain work at its best, giving you the energy to constructively take action. He recommends regularly practicing this skill with the aid of recorded sound timed to cue 6 seconds in and 6 seconds out, which can be set on any commercially available breathing app.

To use coherent breathing:

- Sit or lie comfortably.
- Breathe in on one tone and out on the next.
- Don't feel the need to completely fill your lungs or to squeeze them out.
- When your mind wanders, come back to feeling the breath moving in and out through the nose and throat.
- Ideally practice 3–5 minutes at a time as often as needed.

Touch

Gently putting a hand on her chest and belly as she breathes can also help Keisha compose herself. Physical support from a loved one is another fabulous way to reduce fear and stress. Research shows that a 20-second hug along with 10 minutes of hand-holding can lower your response to stress and anxiety.

Thought Cues

Self-Talk

Giving yourself encouraging messages can help you throw yourself into the idea that you can manage and take action. It's important for Keisha to believe she *can* get to her doctor's office. Research shows that the most important factor in determining our response to pressure is our view of our ability to handle it.

See if it's possible to talk to yourself like a loving, reassuring friend who believes in you. Try to be your own best cheerleader. Some people find it helpful to remind themselves of other difficult obstacles they've been able to face. Remember that you also have new ideas of ways to cope and encourage yourself to use them.

Consider saying:

Just because I'm scared doesn't mean I can't cope.

I have strength and courage, even if it feels hidden.

Sitting with the unknown is hard, but I can get through this.

I wish I didn't have this stress, but I can handle the pressure and rise to the challenge.

I'm learning skills that help me cope.

The butterflies in my stomach are a message that I need to take action about something that is important to me.

My pounding heart is my body's way of giving me energy and courage to meet this challenge and access my strength.

We do realize that self-talk is easier said than done, so keep the conversation going. The more you tell yourself you can cope, the more likely it is that you can actually do it. Marsha likes to say if the salespeople can sell things, you can sell yourself on your courage and strength. We particularly love the Zen wisdom that says when you act as if you always have had courage and strength, you will find you actually do have it.

Dialectical Strategies

Thinking dialectically by including the opposite view offers a more balanced perspective. Keisha can acknowledge that she is scared and still keep in mind that her apprehension is only one part of a bigger picture of herself. Her full story also includes the opposite of fear, her courage. I love the story about the astronaut who says that courage is not about ignoring fear but doing what you need to do even as you feel the fear. Keisha's bravery may feel hidden right now. Yet her ability to recognize that she does indeed also have courage can help her push from the frightened end of her seesaw to the other side so she can throw herself into getting to the doctor's office. Acknowledging both her fear and her bravery can help her support her belief in her capacity to cope.

A fuller perspective about stress can also be very valuable. Naturally no one wants stress. Yet one of the biggest misconceptions is the judgment that stress is only destructive. Indeed the full story about stress is that it both threatens *and* challenges you. Have you noticed that when you feel stressed you work harder to solve your problems and may be motivated to reach out for help? Although we would happily pass on the opportunity, stressful situations can be what my sister likes to call AFGOs (another frigging growth opportunity).

Research shows that a fuller and more balanced view that considers both the upside and downside of stress empowers people to take control of how they respond. People who see the challenge as well as the threat of stress have been shown to be more likely to trust themselves to handle the situation and rise to the challenge. Their resilience actually increases. In addition they show less anxiety, depression, and insomnia as well as more focus, engagement, collaboration, and productivity at work. What's more, the negative health impacts of stress may be minimized.

Coping Ahead

The more you practice dealing with fear, the more confidence you'll have that you can cope. With this skill you rehearse in your mind how to deal with the thing you're afraid of doing. This is useful when you feel unsure of your ability to handle a situation. You make a plan for how you'll manage and imagine what actions you'll take. Deciding which tactics you can constructively use helps you see that there can be a way to move forward without feeling so out of control or blindsided by your emotions. When you have a plan for dealing with unknowns and *what ifs*, you're less likely to feel that it's your job to worry. You can have a greater sense of having some mastery over the way you manage the situation.

Coping ahead has been effective for many people. The steps to follow are:

- Describe the specific situation that is likely to prompt distress
- Name the threat in the situation
- Check the facts
- Imagine the situation in your mind as vividly as possible
- Rehearse coping effectively
- Practice relaxation *after* rehearsing

Let's imagine how Keisha might practice coping ahead. The first thing she needs to do is to describe the situation prompting her distress, which is going to the doctor and anticipating difficult news. Next she names the threat she feels. Keisha had created an entire story about what the news would be and how anxiously she would react. She thought she would be told she needed chemo and would lose her hair. She was afraid that she would feel so distraught that she would break down in front of the doctor.

It's important to be specific about the danger, as the threat of the same situation varies among individuals. For Keisha, that threat was of hair loss, based on her belief that it would be an indication of how seriously unwell she was. To another person the threat of losing her hair from chemo represents a lack of control over the privacy about her illness. This second individual may feel that hair loss is a visible sign that she has cancer. Without hair, she feels that people will be more likely to ask personal questions. Yet for a third person, the threat is that she will not look her best. This individual prides herself on her attractiveness and worries she will no longer have her good looks or be appealing to others.

The next step is to check the facts to see the likelihood of the anticipated threat actually happening. Keisha had a lot of assumptions and ideas about what the doctor would say. She believed that hair loss during chemo came from being so sick from cancer. After checking the facts, she realized that, among other misconceptions, she was conflating worry about treatment side effects with worry about the course of her illness. The fact is that hair loss is not an indication of the virulence of cancer.

Keisha's goal is to use as much detail as possible so she can picture herself in the situation. She decides to use her skills to name and acknowledge her emotions. In addition to being frightened, is she sad? Angry? Embarrassed? She recognizes that she is both sad and angry that she needs treatment at all. She is embarrassed about being so afraid.

Keisha also practices mindfully paying attention to her ideas, judgments, and bodily sensations. She rehearses coping by imagining what unproductive thoughts she might have, such as "I won't be able to cope. I will be too panicked"; "I will embarrass myself if I'm too emotional in front of the doctor"; "I'm just a Nervous Nellie."

She tries to anticipate what new problems could come up. She takes particular notice of how she might avoid her feelings, such as saying "I'm just going to take a nap and not go. I can reschedule this appointment for another day when I feel stronger." She rehearses asking her wise mind whether this behavior is in her interest.

Keisha then decides exactly what actions she might take and what she can say. She makes a list of all the questions she wants to ask the doctor. To help her take action, she imagines calming her anxiety in the waiting room by using coherent breath and/or paired muscle relaxation and reviews the steps to take.

In Chapter 7 we go into detail about effective communication techniques, including using an even tone of voice. Keisha rehearses some of these strategies. She tries to think through what follow-up issues she wants to raise if she needs chemo and will lose her hair. She decides she wants to both ask concrete questions about managing hair loss and raise concerns about the larger health implications. She imagines whom she might ask to go to the doctor with her and what kind of encouragement she might ask them to give her. She talks to people who have lost their hair. She asks a friend if she might be willing to take her to look at wigs if that is necessary.

Imagining a stressful situation can be upsetting, so Keisha then practices paced breathing with a longer exhale to calm herself. Don't forget, you can practice these steps just like Keisha has done.

Short-Term Ways to Tolerate Intense Distress

What can you do when you feel too frightened to hold it together or use any skills and you still need to cope? When your anxiety is above 80 on a scale of 1–100 and wise mind tells you that continuing to pay attention to your fear is no longer in your interest, it can be effective to temporarily shift your attention. Taking your mind off the stressor helps to alter your physiology.

We offer a variety of recommendations as "different strokes work for different folks." Some of the ideas may already be part of your wise mind natural inclination to take care of yourself. We also suggest ways to quiet fearful anxious ideas that are keeping you up at night.

Distraction

The goal at this time is to do things to stir up emotions that are the opposite of what you're feeling. Watch a comedy. Be with your funniest, least serious friend. Be very loud when you sing that silly song. Even better, get your friend to sing with you.

Try your best to immerse yourself as fully as possible in the activity. Effective distraction activities can be quite individual, so choose the activity that is absorbing for you. Swimming is my medicine. I went straight to the pool after coming home with my diagnosis. Others choose different exercise, although this may be a time in your life when you change your exercise regime. Some people can immerse themselves in a puzzle, focusing on the shapes of the pieces, the colors, and where the pieces go. For others, music is the key. Sailing, cleaning, making, building, taking your dog for a walk—do what works for you. Whatever you choose, fully throw yourself into the experience. Feel the wind on your face on that sailboat; tack a few extra times. Take a route that might be new for you. People living with cancer find reading can go both ways—some find it absorbing; others find they have more trouble concentrating at this time.

You also want to choose a distraction strategy that is appropriate for the setting. Indeed, it may not fit your personality or the moment to break into a loud silly song in the doctor's waiting room. We have more options for you.

At certain times, distracting thoughts work better than distracting actions. You want to occupy your mind to keep it from going to anxious worry. You might try naming everything you see and hear that is right in front of you. You can name all the colors in a painting or an actual scene in front of you. You might name textures and materials. "The couch is plaid. The counter is made of Formica." Or try to literally name every object in front of you: "*People* magazine is on the coffee table." Your goal is to keep yourself in the present, avoiding things associated with your worry. When your mind slips back into worry, go back to naming.

Some people find counting things in front of them even more effective. Consider counting the number of people in the waiting room or bricks on the wall. One person did well counting drops from the IV line even though that was something associated with the worry. You might also want to try counting backwards from 100 to 0 to keep your mind occupied. For some, repeating lyrics of a song is effective. One woman sang, "Let It Go" from *Frozen* to herself over and over!

Other people find it useful to try to compartmentalize their anxiety. Some describe putting an imaginary wall around the time and way they worry. They may try to keep certain times of day they allow themselves to agonize. One person found it helpful to use a diary to journal her concerns. The writing helped her name the worries and put them aside.

Another person had a literal "box of burdens" where she could deposit her written concerns and then return the box to the shelf. Some like to imagine a beloved person (grandparent) or spiritual figure (Jesus, God, the Buddha) holding their troubles for them. One other man found it useful to symbolically fill a pitcher of water with his troubles and at least temporarily get rid of them by flushing them down the toilet.

Insomnia

If you're having trouble sleeping, you're not alone. One study reports that up to 80% of cancer patients have sleep problems during treatment. Sleep disruption may come from medication and/or stress and anxiety. Watch out for middle-of-the-night thinking, when worries may seem even more catastrophic than in the daytime. It is useful to remind yourself that often those thoughts are less catastrophic in the morning.

Some people find they may take up to a half hour or so to fall asleep. Do your best to avoid panicking about not sleeping. While the anxiety about not sleeping and its impact are stressful, the worry only perpetuates the insomnia. Marsha finds it very effective to count to get to sleep and has her whole family doing so. The key to Marsha's strategy is to notice your doubt about the effectiveness of counting and your wish to quit, but keep counting. Do not give up or decide you just can't sleep at all.

FIVE

Managing Sadness

If you're feeling sad right now, you're not alone. No one is happy to have cancer. People can understandably feel down if they believe they are losing or have lost something meaningful. Would you expect someone else in your situation not to feel sad?

In this chapter we offer a fuller perspective on sadness and consider the value of grieving. We review skills to help you accept your feelings and present ways to reduce them when they get too intense. We introduce additional coping strategies and ways to give you time away from being so sad.

Sadness and Grieving with Cancer

As you may expect, if people feel they are losing their health or parts of their body, or they can't take part in activities that are important to them, they may feel very sad. Some may also mourn the loss of future opportunities or a changed self-definition. Let's look at the story of Maria, who is in despair that cancer surgery may also impact her fertility.

Like Maria, many people fight the feeling and tell themselves not to be sad. The wish to stay away from extreme sadness is totally understandable. Intense sadness is painful. Some judge sadness as a weakness. Or they might assume that, if they allow themselves to cry, their strong feelings may never go away. They may even start believing they will never be happy again or their unhappiness will drive loved ones away. Of course, believing these things doesn't make them true.

The fact is that if profound sadness, sometimes called *grief*, comes up, it can't be avoided. Indeed, you're less likely to remain sad if you **allow the emotion to come and then allow it to pass by making sure you're not holding or intensifying the feeling.** Recall the open-palm image. Let's try to understand this advice.

Many people have found that grieving helps them acknowledge a loss and return to functioning more normally. The grieving process involves accepting what has happened and paying attention to the experience of the tragedy, including allowing extreme sadness. Acknowledging the emotion is an essential step.

Sadness can facilitate constructive grief. When people are sad, they instinctively turn inward. They withdraw. They slow down. They take a forced time-out to recognize what's happened and fully consider what to do next. Studies show sad people become more self-perceptive.

Sadness can also deepen relationships. When people feel sad, they look sad. Their appearance elicits sympathy and sends a compelling message that connection and support are needed. Research shows that sorrow also helps build compassion and empathy. Sad people some-times become more thoughtful and less biased in their perceptions of others.

On the other hand, grieving is difficult and can take you into vul-nerable territory. It demands bravely facing painful realities. It means not turning away from intense feelings despite the fear of remaining sad. Maria's moments of despair can seem like depression when she feels angry, lonely, anxious, irritable, or helpless as well as having changes in her sleep, energy, appetite, or concentration. Yet there are important differences. When the reaction is limited to grief, those depression-like reactions may not necessarily last a long time. Despite periods of pro-found sadness, Maria can still find some moments of happiness and vital-ity.

In fact, ongoing depression is less likely when sad feelings are allowed to ebb and flow naturally. Indeed, there are ways to accept that sadness has come up and also let it pass by in its own time. Let's look at how Maria tries to be aware of whether she is holding on to or building up sad feelings.

Observe to Assess and Control Sadness

Many of the strategies already presented are very valuable in both supporting constructive grief and reducing unconstructive sadness. They are not magic bullets that always get rid of intense sadness but can help to minimize the feelings. Studies show that people using mindfulness skills often advance more quickly through the initial stages of mourning and demonstrate significant reductions in depression and anxiety.

Although easier said than done, pausing to pay attention to her experience can help Maria assess and manage her despair. Ensuring that the intensity of her emotion makes sense and noticing the distinction between allowing her sadness and increasing it can help her decide whether it is in her interest to try to decrease her sadness.

The ideal **steps to reduce sadness are:**

- Acknowledge the loss by pausing to observe
  - Allow and name the feeling
  - Detect where and how the emotion is expressed in your body
  - Notice thoughts
- Check the facts
- Use dialectical strategies
- Ask wise mind

Maria feels overwhelmed by the prospect of stopping to intentionally notice her experience. Thinking about the reality of her life right now feels intolerable. She wishes there was a way to get around her unavoidable feelings. She doesn't want to acknowledge a truth that can stir up unbearable sadness. Is this process really going to be helpful? She worries despair will take over.

On the other hand, she has been told that refusing to acknowledge the truth of her situation and how she feels about it can keep her stuck in unhappiness and other painful emotions. She is not sure she can do all these steps but realizes that the more of them she does, the better off she is likely to be.

Notice and Name Feelings

Since Maria can't stop her feelings, she decides that she may as well try to control them by acknowledging them. Keeping "name it to tame it" (Chapter 4) in mind, she remembers that labeling emotions lowers their intensity. She reluctantly tries to do her best to allow and recognize her distraught feelings.

It's not easy for Maria to figure out what she is feeling. As is not unusual, Maria's sadness is initially blocked by anger. She recognizes her heartache and anguish only after the anger passes.

This list of some of the most common words used to identify sadness is a useful guide to help Maria recognize and name sad feelings.

Agony	Discontentment	Melancholy
Alienation	Dismay	Misery
Alone	Displeasure	Neglect
Anguish	Distress	Pity
Crushed	Gloom	Rejection
Defeat	Glumness	Sadness
Dejection	Grief	Sorrow
Depression	Homesickness	Suffering
Despair	Hurt	Unhappiness
Disappointment	Insecurity	Woe
Disconnectedness	Loneliness	

Pay Attention to Bodily Sensations

Maria can also recognize sadness by noticing how it feels in her body. "Grief is registered in our sinews and muscles," said Francis Weller in *The Wild Edge of Sorrow*. "It feels labored, as though a great weight has settled on our chest or heaviness has entered our bones. We know grief by its felt experience; it is tangible. It is here, in our sighing and sensing body, that we encounter the terrain of sorrow."

Sadness can dampen physiological functioning. Some people are more lethargic. Their heart rate may be down. Their physical stance may sag. They may speak more slowly.

When Maria pauses to pay attention, she is aware of the heaviness and hollow feeling in her chest. She tries to notice any sensations behind her eyes, shoulders, belly, and throat. She attempts to observe whether her face is sagging, her eyebrows are pinched together, or her eyes drooping. She sees that her jaw is slackening and realizes her lower lip is drawn out in a pout. She is sobbing. She notices that she is speaking in a quiet, slow, monotonous voice. She is aware of how lethargic she feels. She recognizes that she is slumping. She tries to detect whether her sadness has disrupted her normal appetite, digestion, or sleep.

Notice Thoughts That May Increase Sadness

Sad people can make negative judgments and assumptions about themselves, their coping, and their relationships. Some even decide they deserve what has happened, which, of course, is rarely true. Unfavorable self-judgments, blame, and ruminating ideas only increase their misery.

Maria has always seen herself as an attractive, fulfilled, competent woman with a plan to have children in the future. Now she questions whether she will still be attractive if she loses her hair during treatment. Will removing her ovaries make her less of a woman? Can she still be a biological mother? Is she now defective?

She imagines others either do or should pity her. She judges her intense grief as self-indulgence and starts referring to herself as "Debbie Downer," a person even she wants to avoid. She starts to believe Debbie Downer is her new permanent identity. She is having so much trouble tolerating her own despondent feelings that she assumes others cannot stand the pain either and may be driven away. She considers trying to keep her feelings to herself, yet the idea only intensifies her sense of isolation.

Check the Facts

Next, Maria tries to gather more information to make certain that both her factual and emotional assumptions are correct. She wants to be sure she is not making herself sadder with unverified judgmental ideas about herself, her coping, or her interactions with others. Is she misunderstanding medical facts, believing unproven assumptions, or grieving over possibilities that may not even happen?

Checking the facts can help Maria assess whether there is as much of a threat as she imagines. She is assuming that she won't be able to cope, that her relationships may be compromised by her appearance or sadness, and that she can never bear children. It is not clear that any of these assumptions are accurate. She explores whether the medical reality is that her loss is actually the ability to have children when and how she planned. She tries to find out whether freezing her eggs and carrying a child at a later date is a possibility for her.

Dialectical Strategies

Maria uses dialectical strategies to recall that **sadness is part of a bigger picture that includes the opposite view.** She tries to keep the seesaw metaphor in mind, remembering that when there is motion between the two sides of the full story one is less likely to be stuck in despair. She attempts to remember that, although moments of joy feel hidden right now, life includes moments of both deep sadness *and* profound joy.

Although it is not easy, she does her best to take a more balanced perspective and avoid viewing things in black-or-white extremes. She considers whether the most complete story of herself includes sides of her she is now overlooking. Is she more capable of coping than she thinks? Does having children in a different time frame or way than she has hoped or imagined actually mean she is defective or worthless? Is that reality her only defining characteristic? She tries to keep a fuller perspective in mind, recognizing that different does not mean defective or worthless.

Wise Mind

Maria **asks her wise mind whether the intensity of her emotion is in her interest or she wants to make changes to reduce her sadness.** Does she have a constructive balance between denying her sorrow and letting those feelings take over? She doesn't want to invalidate her understandable grief. Yet her new medical reality and intense emotions do not have to define her. Has she unproductively assumed she will never be happy again? Is she narrowing her perspective and discounting positive parts of herself and her life that can bring her happiness? She reminds herself to do her best to take that helicopter view for a bigger picture that can help her have a balanced wise mind perspective. She recognizes that her sorrow makes sense but she may be sadder than is in her interest. She decides to try to reduce the intensity of her feelings. Let's look at some ways others have found helpful that she can consider using.

Opposite Action for Sadness

With this strategy you do your best to **try to think and act in ways that are opposite to the tendency to withdraw from others, helplessly and hopelessly giving up thinking, doing, or pushing for things that can make you feel better.** The goal is to **balance these unproductive inclinations** by building up pleasant, optimistic feelings and experiences. People have found that this approach helps them move away from a physical and/ or emotional slump by putting emphasis and weight on the other side of the pessimistic, unhappy end of the seesaw. While easier said than done, the idea is to make a change to the negative feedback loop by thinking, acting, and/or cueing your body in a different way.

We do want to be clear here that we are not simply suggesting that you "be positive." Well-meaning prescriptions to "think and act positive" can unwittingly trivialize grief and distress. It is natural that you may feel sad or think about the ways life is not going the way you want and need at this time.

On the other hand, the most complete view does also include positive parts. You are alive. The sun still shines. People care about you. Ruminating about an unhappy state of affairs without also bringing upbeat thoughts to mind or doing pleasurable things can throw you out of balance. Happy parts of life and encouraging signs can easily be missed.

Rebalancing is not easy. The negativity bias tips the weight to the pessimistic side, and negative thoughts stick like Velcro. You are doing the best you can. Yet you also have the choice to try to make changes to restore the balance. Studies show the effort may be worth it. A fuller, balanced perspective fosters resilience. What's more, building up positive feelings can reduce the likelihood of depression and strengthen the immune system.

Let's consider what changes to your thoughts, your body, and/or your actions may put more weight on the opposite side of staying so sad. We present a lot of options. Choose the ones that seem good for you, and don't give yourself a hard time if you're not doing them all.

Positive Thoughts

Can you try to pay attention to see whether you're forgetting or overlooking anything positive? Is it possible to recall wonderful memories? At times people may be afraid to be optimistic and disregard encouraging indications. Are you discounting positive signs that might give you hope? Look at how you're trying to improve your coping.

Self-Talk

Many find it valuable to use encouraging thoughts to help them believe in themselves and their ability to cope. See if you can give yourself a supportive pep talk to help you stop thinking you can't deal with what is happening and can't make changes. Consider saying:

> I can cope even though I worry that I can't.
>
> My sadness is understandable, and it's unlikely I will be this sad forever.
>
> I can do my best not only to pay attention to what makes me sad but also to try to notice the positive parts of my life.
>
> I can make an effort to use some helpful coping strategies. Even more important, I can give myself credit for how hard I'm trying without giving up.

Marsha particularly loves this last one and personally finds giving herself credit for not quitting extremely helpful.

You will have to repeat these things over and over again. Yet, when you say them often enough, you may begin to believe them, feel better, and do something differently.

Gratitude

In the words of Francis Weller, "We cannot possibly face the horrors . . . with any sense of balance without also remembering the beauty of the world—the plum blossoms and mustard blooming. We must couple grief and gratitude in a way that encourages us to stay open to life."

When you feel so unlucky, it may feel like too much to ask to also keep in mind and appreciate positive moments and upbeat people. On the other hand, research shows that at least trying to acknowledge any blessing may be worth your while. In one study, patients who made a weekly list of five things for which they were grateful felt significantly happier and reported fewer health problems than groups that focused on hassles or only wrote about ordinary events. One man told me that if he ignored the good things in life he spent the whole day unhappy and lost the day. He decided that a little good is better than no good, even if he got 5% of the day.

Are you open to deciding to pause to be sure you don't miss that beautiful sunset? Can you take a moment to recognize caring support of the people who are trying to help you—a helpful doctor, nurse, or loving family member? Are you aware of how you feel when someone makes special efforts for you? That man found it helpful to be sure he didn't miss extra touches they provided for his comfort at his chemo center. He made an effort to notice the thoughtfully considered snacks and the comfy blankets.

While it may seem difficult, is it possible to also pay attention to and appreciate any positive things that are still a part of your life? Dinesh, the young man introduced in Chapter 1, said that thinking how much worse things could be made him grateful for what remained. He realized how lucky he felt to have hair after being told he would eventually be bald from the chemo.

Be sure not to give yourself a hard time when your mind naturally wanders to the negative. Those inevitable judgments will come up. Perhaps you even wonder whether you deserve anything positive or worry how much more might be expected of you if you feel happier. Do your best to remember how natural your feelings are and refocus your attention to also include positive thoughts.

Bodily Cues for Change

There are a number of different physical changes you can make in order to feel differently. The idea here is to boost your depressed energy level, posture, speech, and/or heart rate. **Anything you are considering should be reviewed with your health care provider first.**

Physical Exercise

Discuss with your doctor whether there is a safe way for you to get your heart rate up.

Breath

Many people have found their breath to be a valuable tool to energize themselves. Consider trying a breathing strategy called **Ha breath,** described by Dr. Richard Brown, author of *The Healing Power of Breath*:

- Do your best to energize your mind and body.
- Stand up tall, elbows bent, palms facing up.
- As you inhale, draw your elbows back behind you, palms continuing to face up.
- Then exhale quickly and thrust your palms forward, turning them downward while saying "Ha" out loud.
- Repeat quickly 15 to 20 times.
- Rest for 30 seconds noting changes in your body, thoughts and breath.
- Repeat for more energy.

Posture

See if it is at all possible to take a positive body stance, using a "bright" body posture, with head up, eyes open, and shoulders back, speaking in an upbeat voice. You might even consider trying to slightly turn the corners of your mouth upward in a half smile.

Pleasurable Sensations

Your body can also be a wonderful source of pleasure. Consider the ways your five senses may help to change your mood.

Tasting: Eat or drink some of your favorite things. What about sampling a special treat you like to eat or drink—fresh-squeezed fruit juice, special baked goods, or childhood favorites?

Seeing: Do you get particular enjoyment from seeing something beautiful? Perhaps watching children or animals at play brings you great joy. Take in the splendor of nature. Try not to miss a bright-blue sky. Savor pleasing art. Relish that dance performance.

Touching: Would it feel delightful to you to wrap yourself in a blanket or put creamy lotion on your body? Maybe a warm bath or massage brings you pleasure. Perhaps the wind on your face or hugging someone brings you the greatest happiness.

Hearing: Consider listening to or playing invigorating music. Are the sounds of nature or happy children particularly uplifting to you?

Smelling: Do you enjoy the aroma of certain foods? Maybe the smell of a scented candle, incense, or a special cologne or aftershave is especially appealing. Are the fresh smells of nature more pleasing to you?

Do what is most pleasant for you!

Actions

One of the best ways to rebalance is to decrease behavior that makes you sadder and increase behavior that makes you happier. Even if you have to talk yourself into it, try your best to *do* more enjoyable things.

Pleasant Events

It may not be easy, but see if you can take time to do at least one thing each day that brings you pleasure. The more pleasurable it is, the more it can take you away from sadness. It can be a pleasant activity or time with someone special. Do your best to stay open to others and let them know the connection is important to you. Savor even the smallest daily events.

Laughter

While laughing may seem out of place when you feel so down, humor can be a terrific way to balance sadness. The wisdom of this strategy is expressed in the wise saying "Laughter is the best medicine." Humor helps to make grief bearable and has been reported to boost mood, strengthen immune system functioning, diminish pain, and protect against damaging effects of stress. Sincere laughing and smiling are contagious and encourage more pleasant connections with others. Research shows that cracking a grin when the chips are down improves long-term coping. The more grieving people laughed and smiled in the early months of a loss, the better their mental health was over the next 2 years.

I wish I had taken a more lighthearted attitude earlier in my treatment. It took a while for me to realize that joking did not necessarily deny the seriousness of my situation. One friend taught me how her gleeful hysterics in considering an orange Mohawk at the wig store reduced her sense of helplessness and despair about her hair falling out. Dinesh told me, "I want and need to thank Jon Stewart for helping me through cancer." He spent every day watching *The Daily Show*, every episode of *30 Rock*, and any other comedy he could find. Another man described how helpful the slapstick of Laurel and Hardy was to him.

How can you bring humor into your life? Crack jokes; watch funny movies. Listen to humorous stories. Ask people around you or online to help you find funny jokes or memes. Try to hang around with people who have a good sense of humor—even if you might have to sometimes tell them that some jokes are not helpful to you.

Building Mastery

Activities that increase your belief that you're still competent and have the capacity to control your own life can also be a way to help you feel less helpless and hopeless. You may not be able to do all of the things you used to be able to do, but that doesn't mean you can't do anything. Do your best to avoid telling yourself that you're helpless and can't do anything. If you can open your eyes, you can do something. As difficult as this might seem, mastery has been shown to increase resistance to being depressed.

Try your best to use self-talk to encourage yourself to try to do things that make you feel more capable and self-confident. We have found it useful to try to plan on doing at least one thing each day to build a sense of accomplishment. Try something challenging but not ridiculously out of the question.

Plan for success, not failure. Gradually increase the difficulty over time. If the first job is too difficult, do something a little easier next time. If the challenge is too easy, try something a little harder next time. It can be new challenges each day or a series of tasks that help you develop skill in a new area.

Dinesh decided to hone his cooking skills during a time he was too unwell to be at college. One day he would teach himself how to dice an onion. Another day he tried poaching an egg. He developed a sense of competence and learned to make the protein-rich foods he needed to build up his strength. His cooking became one of the most expressive things he did.

Journaling

Another activity that people have found valuable is to keep a journal. Some have described the way writing about an experience of loss helps to name and process overwhelming feelings. Cancer patients whose writing includes positives were found to have lower physical symptom reports and fewer medical appointments. Additional studies show the way writing about joyful experiences enhances positive mood.

Contributing

Yet another way to balance sad feelings is to do things for others. Indeed, multiple studies have shown that the more people feel like they are helping others, the less depressed they feel.

Dinesh, the budding chef, eventually began hosting dinner parties. His hobby became a way to connect to and give back to friends who were supporting him. A woman used needlepoint in much the same way. Her needlework became an important vehicle to create enduring things for her loved ones. Another man said that a good day is when he does something fun, learns something, or helps someone else. Not everyone is able to volunteer at the local food pantry as he does. Yet you may want to consider reaching out or helping someone else, doing something thoughtful, or giving something away. Some people find that supporting fellow patients benefits them both.

Next we turn to managing anger.

SIX

Managing Anger

Anybody can be angry—that is easy, but to be angry with the right person and to the right degree and at the right time and for the right purpose and in the right way . . . is not easy.

—ARISTOTLE

As we have seen, people respond to cancer in many different ways. Being aware of your own reactions is key. If you notice you're angry, you're not alone.

Is your anger constructive? Do your feelings let you or others know that there is a problem? Perhaps your anger expresses your frustration about being in physical and/or emotional pain. Does the emotion motivate you to take care of yourself or help you get what you need? Does it help you avoid other uncomfortable feelings, feel less vulnerable, or minimize self-criticism?

Maybe, on the other hand, you worry that your anger is destructive. Do you criticize yourself for your feelings? Are you concerned that your emotion is out of control or may damage relationships? Do you want to reduce your anger?

Recall that emotions are **not** necessarily constructive *or* destructive. Anger can range in intensity from mild irritation to rage and fury. At times, some degree of anger can be helpful. On the other hand, overly intense anger can be harmful. **The ideal is to respond to a message to** protect yourself or fight an injustice in a way that does not damage a relationship or how you feel about yourself.

This chapter reviews skills to help you identify what you're feeling and consider whether expressing your emotion at this time is in your best interest. We introduce the **STOP** skill, reemphasizing a distinction between feeling an emotion and taking action. We offer techniques including sensitive self-talk to reduce unproductive anger and introduce **self-soothing strategies to help you tolerate pain and other distressing situations.** Indeed, there are possible ways to get through this tough stuff.

Understanding Anger and Cancer

Cancer can be life threatening. Recall that when your body senses a threat, a fight-flight-or-freeze response can be triggered. Your body's forceful response to the perception of grave danger can also stir up very intense emotion.

Fierce emotion may have been adaptive to spur the caveman to fight off an attacking lion. But in this day and age, it is not clear whom or what to fight to protect you from cancer. Outrage over the limitations of health care providers or modern medicine may not help to ensure your safety. Bitterness at an unjust world or blaming professionals, loved ones, or yourself may appear to offer a sense of control or seem to answer the questions "Why?" or "Why me?" Yet the explanation may come at a cost. Intense hostility may endanger relationships or leave you feeling out of control or ashamed. Occasionally, anger can impact the immune system or worsen pain.

Anger may also be a reaction to the distress of having to endure the losses and the physical and/or emotional pain that may come with cancer. Multiple studies report a link between anger, animosity toward others or oneself, and pain. Perhaps you're angry at not getting the relief or understanding you feel you need. Sometimes others are responsible. At other times you may be facing the frustrating reality that things can't be changed as quickly as you want or need.

Let's take a look at how to use a new skill called STOP and some strategies you already know to help you effectively manage anger.

The STOP Skill

This strategy is an invaluable first step when you are angry. The goal is to **pause to remember a valuable distinction between feeling an emotion and necessarily acting on it.** Your first inclination is not always the most constructive.

> **S: Stop** and try not to act on your feelings without thinking.
>
> **T: Try** to take a deep breath and take a moment before reacting.
>
> **O: Observe** your body and thoughts by noticing as much about the full situation as you can. See if you can be aware of what is happening both inside you and around you.
>
> **P: Proceed** mindfully by asking wise mind if it is useful to express your feelings right now

Do the best you can without giving yourself a hard time. This ideal is easier said than done.

Pay Attention to Your Body

The O of STOP is to observe. See if you can notice where and how anger is expressed in your body. The *fight* of the fight-flight-or-freeze response may have revved up your body to take action. Is your heart pounding? Is your face flushed or hot? Do you notice muscles tightening? Are you clenching your teeth or hands? Frowning? Some people grin or cry when angry. Are you aware of an urge to blow up, hit something, hurt someone, or send an irate e-mail?

Notice Your Feelings

Next see if you can pay attention to your emotions. Your anger can sometimes seem like static on the radio. When you fine-tune your receiver, you may be clearer about your experience.

It may seem like we're all well aware of being angry. Yet at times some chronic pain patients have difficulty recognizing their emotions.

Being aware of some degree of anger can be an important signal that something is amiss and there is a need to take care of yourself. When you ignore feelings, your pain may sometimes be more severe, you may be more upset, or relationships may be compromised.

Mindfulness can also help you consider whether your reaction is stronger than necessary or if you're holding on to feelings that are not constructive. When you're aware of your own experience, you may be less likely to misplace or unproductively intensify your anger. You have the chance to see whether your annoyance is a response to what someone has or has not done or whether you're upset at having to endure such a distressing situation.

Identify Your Emotion

Anger can be labeled in many different ways. It can be useful to know some of the most common words used to identify this emotion. Which labels best describe how you're feeling?

Anger	Ferocity	Outrage
Agitation	Frustration	Rage
Aggravation	Grouchiness	Vengefulness
Annoyance	Grumpiness	Wrath
Bitterness	Hostility	
Exasperation	Indignation	

Recall the motto "Name it to tame it!" Putting a name to the experience helps to quiet the feeling.

Become Aware of Your Thoughts

See if you can keep in mind that "emotions love themselves" and your thoughts can further fuel your anger. One study found that mere anticipation of pain was enough to provoke anger in healthy individuals. Holding on to or feeding irritation can stoke feelings of outrage or fury. Try to remember that each time you identify an angry thought you're mindfully training yourself not to stay with these thoughts.

See if it's possible to pay attention to your assumptions and judgments. Can you notice whether you've narrowed your attention to focus on injustices? Are you thinking about how unfair your situation is? Do you tell yourself that life "should be" different? Are you ruminating about the original situation that made you angry or recalling additional things that have gone wrong in the past? Are you imagining future situations that may yet go wrong?

Try to pay attention to whether you're judging yourself for feeling agitated. A young mother in a lot of pain gave herself a terrible time for feeling impatient with her children. Have you decided that any degree of anger is destructive? I felt critical of myself for how satisfying I found my indignation about some people's reactions to my cancer. I assumed a "bigger" person would not be as annoyed or self-righteous as I was. Have you ever felt this way?

Perhaps you notice that you're worried that if you acknowledge any form of anger you will automatically act on it. One woman was concerned that admitting her ire would change how she was in the world and how she felt about herself. She said, "I was raised to be a lady and grateful, but this sucks. I know it is no one's fault, but I am not happy about how tired I am. I don't want to have a negative, angry attitude, but it is exasperating that people don't get how incredibly difficult it is for me."

Check the Facts

Try to examine your assumptions and check the facts to see whether you may be intensifying your emotions. **Blame is an idea that empowers anger.** Are you holding yourself, someone else, or something responsible for things that may not be in anyone's control?

Wise Mind

Do your best to pause to ask wise mind whether the strength of your anger makes sense in this situation. Do you have a constructive balance between recognizing a message to take care of yourself and holding on to those feelings past their usefulness? Is your emotion effective in helping you speak up for yourself? Is the intensity of your anger getting in your way? Can you look at the pros and cons of the way you're coping? One man said his anger at his doctor made him feel stronger and gave him a villain that motivated him to work harder. He also considered whether the risk of compromising an important relationship was worth the trade-off of feeling less vulnerable. I had to ask myself if my own indignation was helpful or worth my critical self-judgment.

A wise mind does not see things as one way *or* the other. It's possible that this man's feelings, like my own, arose for understandable reasons, our criticisms made sense, *and* we might also have wanted to try to reduce our anger. Can we find a middle ground between staying silent and attacking? Our goal is to take care of ourselves *and* reduce the emotion. Indeed, in Chapter 7 we offer ways to assert your needs *and* protect your relationships.

Let's look at a way to decrease the strength of feelings that might not be in your interest right now.

Opposite Action for Anger

The goal of this strategy is to act opposite of the angry urge to be aggressive, overly critical, and alienating. You try your best to be a little bit nicer when raising concerns.

When you're angry, you're often physiologically aroused, tense, and can have indignant thoughts. Making changes to your body and thoughts may help to rebalance the feedback loop, minimizing the urge to be overtly hostile.

Physical Changes

As with every physical strategy, check with your doctor first. With medical approval you might try to **bring down your physical arousal by changing your breathing, body tension, and/or temperature. Paced breathing** (see page 45) can be used to change your respiration. Recall that this skill can reduce your level of arousal and promote calm. Relaxing may help you feel less annoyed.

Paired muscle relaxation (see page 45) is also an excellent way to reduce physical tension and promote calm.

In addition, **physical exercise** can help you calm down when you're revved up by emotion. However, this may not be the time in your life for intense exercise. Ask your doctor if there is a safe way for you to burn stored-up energy. If your situation allows, even a gentle walk can sometimes help you feel and think differently.

The following technique to lower your **body temperature** can be helpful if your feelings are too intense and you need to calm down quickly. Again, be sure to **check with your medical provider before trying this,** as very cold water decreases your heart rate.

> To reduce your body temperature:
>
> - Put your full face into cold water or hold a cold ice pack (plastic ziplock bag of ice or cold water) on your eyes and cheeks.
>
> - Keep the water above 50° Fahrenheit and avoid ice if you are allergic to cold.
>
> - Hold your breath for 15–30 seconds.
>
> - Your heart rate should now slow down, reducing blood flow to nonessential organs while redirecting it to your brain and heart.

Changes in Your Thoughts

You are likely to be as rigid in your thinking as you are in your body. Loosening strident beliefs may help you think more flexibly. Your assumptions and judgments may not all be correct.

See if you can keep **dialectical strategies** in mind and pause to remember that there is always another side to your ideas. It's helpful for the young mother who feels guilty about being impatient with her children to remember that her situation is too complex to say *either* that her children are to blame *or* she is a selfish, insensitive mother. A more balanced view can help her avoid identifying with only one negative part of the story. When she thinks about both sides, she realizes a more complete reality. "In the day pain medication makes me too drowsy to be sufficiently responsive to the kids." Yet she is exhausted after being up all night in an "unrelenting shit storm," clawing at herself from a reaction to medication. Can she balance her critical self-judgments by remembering that agitation is a common response to physical and emotional distress? Considering the opposite side may help her realize that she may *both* be irritated *and* want to reduce her anger to be responsive to her children's clamor for her attention. Indeed she may recall that an inner feeling of agitation is not the same as outwardly expressing rage.

Are you reducing the situation to right *or* wrong? I was chagrined to realize that I may have been spending more energy fighting to prove I was right than solving my problem. The man who thought his anger at his doctor motivated him to work harder wanted to believe the problem could be as simple as one of them trying harder. Painfully, sometimes responding effectively to one's needs is more complex.

When you expand your views to **include someone else's perspective,** you can shake up narrow thinking. Stepping into another's shoes sometimes helps to reduce anger. Recall how Sara was less upset after she considered reasons other than her doctor's insensitivity that may have kept her from returning Sara's call as expected. Try your best to consider what parts of your story might be missing to look at the fullest picture.

Self-Soothing

At times you may be frustrated or irritated by an insufficient response to your emotional or physical distress. Sometimes the people around you or the universe can't give you what you want and need.

Self-soothing can be a useful way to calm or relax yourself if you need to find a way to tolerate distress when things cannot be changed right away. The strategy here is to take kind and gentle care of yourself. You try to balance the agitation in your body, the upsetting assumptions, and the self-critical judgments with calming, comforting, sensitive sensations, thoughts, and actions. For some people, taking responsibility for nurturing themselves also brings a greater sense of control.

Let's look at how you can use physical sensations or images to try to soothe yourself.

Self-Soothing with Physical Sensations

Do your best to nurture your body in gentle and comforting ways. The goal is to create pleasant bodily sensations to balance the ways cancer treatment can sometimes be physically harsh and leave your body feeling like an object that is acted upon.

Consider what **touch** might be soothing to you. Do you enjoy a hot bath, massage, lotions, or oils on your body? Are you someone who relishes crisp clean sheets, soft clothes, or feeling snuggly wrapped in a comforting texture? One woman described how petting her cat was the thing that relaxed her most. Taking a plush teddy bear to chemo comforted another person. Another had a small "feely pillow" made out of soft velvet. Choose the touch that works for you. At times, a hug is the most consoling. Consider acting loving toward yourself. You might gently and sensitively bring your hand to your own heart.

What **smells** are pleasant to you? Do you like lavender, vanilla, or fresh-baked bread? Do you have a favorite cologne, shampoo, or aftershave? Does a burning candle or incense cue relaxation for you? Are the scents of fresh air and nature calming and soothing to you? If you can't literally be outside to smell the roses, bring some fresh flowers inside or open the window.

Think about what **sounds** are most relaxing to you. Many people find it useful to have a recording of their favorite music available to listen to at agitating times. For some the music is classical or lullabies. Others find comfort in hearing invigorating sounds. Are you soothed by the sounds of nature? Crashing waves? Chirping birds? Rustling leaves? Rainfall?

Comfort food has become its own category for a good reason. What is your favorite thing to eat? Do your **taste** buds clamor for butterscotch, chocolate ice cream, or other sweets? Is your special treat fresh-squeezed juice, homemade soup, or a cup of tea? If you are nauseous or your palate has changed, it is also possible that taste may not be a soothing sensation right now.

What **images** are most comforting to you? One man described the joy he found in watching the playfulness of his grandchildren. Is it relaxing for you to look at a beautiful book? Do you enjoy viewing fine art or photography? Perhaps you can watch a movie or video of majestic scenery or other pleasant images? Are you someone who finds calm in watching the flame of a candle? For many the most soothing sights are nature, such as the stars at night, a beautiful sunset, or a roaring ocean.

Self-Soothing with Imagery

When comforting sensations are not immediately available or you can't physically be in a calming place, it may still be possible to bring an image of soothing people, places, and situations to mind.

Imagery has been shown to help cancer patients tolerate pain and other distressing situations. The objective is to temporarily turn your attention away from distress by imagining a connection to a person, place, or time in which you have felt calm, safe, and secure.

Consider creating a mental picture of a relaxing place. Soothing images are personal. Some find ease by imagining themselves next to a babbling brook strewn with autumn leaves or a meadow filled with wildflowers. Others find ease in bringing mental pictures of loved ones, including future family, to mind. Choose the image that works for you.

Some people use imagery to find strength by mentally identifying with a powerful image such as a mountain or an inspirational person. The figure may come from a personal relationship or be someone from history, such as Jesus, Moses, Gandhi, the Buddha, or Nelson Mandela.

To use imagery:

- Close your eyes and slow down your breathing, with a longer exhale than inhale.

- See if you can bring to mind a picture of a person, place, or time that evokes safety, ease, or protection. Is your comforting place indoors or outside?

- Do your best to notice the sights, sounds, and sensations of feeling safety and connection by imagining all the details of this special place. Are you alone, or do you have others with you? Are there animals present?

- Focus on all of the beautiful things you see that make your place enjoyable. Is there water or vegetation nearby? What are the colors and shapes of any objects you see?

- Do your best to see if you can let the warmth and friendliness of a smile spread over your body.

- Feel the outer corners of your eyes lift slightly and your flesh soften as if you are smiling into your eyes.

- Let your brow be smooth.

- Feel a real smile at your mouth and sense the inside of your mouth smiling.

- Relax your jaw. Notice the sensations in your mouth and cheek.

- Visualize and feel a smile spread through your heart and chest. Let your smile create space for whatever you are feeling.

- Notice any pleasing tactile sensations such as the temperature. Is the sun on your face, or is there any breeze? Are you touching a surface that brings you comfort? Maybe soft sand or a cozy blanket brings ease to you. If there is an animal present, is it soothing to pet it?

- Try your best to pay attention to any relaxing sounds. Perhaps there is soothing music playing. Do you hear rustling leaves or waves lapping ashore? Are there calming voices of loved ones in the background? Is there something special they are saying?

- See if you can imagine any tastes or pleasing aromas. Is your favorite food being prepared? Can you recall and savor the smells and flavor? Perhaps there are other fragrances that delight you.

- To add further detail to this scene, picture yourself in this peaceful place. Are you sitting, relaxing, and enjoying this calming place, or walking, listening, eating, or doing other activities? Allow your breath to lengthen, to feel comfort and ease. Slow down your exhale to feel more relaxed.

- Notice and name the emotions you feel. Is there calm, relaxation, joy, happiness, or ease?

- Register any thoughts about what it is like to be in this place. See if you can find a message to carry with you that goes with feelings of ease and safety. Explore whispering the words to yourself.

- Try your best to remember all the details of this special place and time so you can re-create the experience of safety and connection.

- Know that you can return to this peaceful place by recalling the picture in your mind during distressing times when you need to relax and regroup.

Self-Care Can Be a Challenge

At times people can be uncomfortable caring for themselves. Some may be angry that the world has disappointed them and they have to do their own caretaking. Others believe that being gentle to themselves will make them sadder or weaker or make them feel sorry for themselves, undermining their will to take responsibility for themselves. One woman said, "I am not sure what is worse—being a bitch or having a pity party." Yet research has shown that self-compassion actually strengthens and motivates one to be proactive.

Sometimes people need to use opposite action to be kind to themselves. They may believe they don't deserve kind care. One young unmarried woman had a bilateral mastectomy and lost her fertility but said she had no right to complain because others had tougher chemo regimens than she did.

Some can feel they have done something wrong. They may feel ashamed or unworthy of sensitive care. Like me, they may give themselves a hard time if they feel short-tempered with people who may be trying to be helpful. Recall the young mother who overly simplified her situation and decided that if the children were right to want her attention, then there must be something wrong with her for not giving them the attention they deserve. Others are angry with themselves and may exaggerate their responsibility for changing or their capacity to alter how their body responds and its impact on their family. They may tyrannize themselves, believing the course of their illness is due to a failure of will or another moral or character flaw. The list of things that they "should" do better can be exhaustive and exhausting!

"Eat healthier."

"Be stronger."

"Sleep more."

"Be more positive."

"Fight harder."

"Be less emotional and stressed."

"Exercise more."

The fact is that many factors go to into surviving cancer. Variables such as genetics, the environment, and luck are completely outside your control. Indeed, there is little consistent evidence that a mindset such as a fighting spirit, hopelessness, helplessness, denial, or avoidance impacts cancer survival or recurrence.

On the other hand, we all have regrets about things we did or didn't do. Undeniably, there may be times that honest assessment does include facing some accountability for distressing facts. Ron, a lifelong smoker, has to come to terms with the impact of his smoking on his lung cancer without allowing a toxic layer of self-disgust to cloud his view of the most complete picture. His smoking is one of many facets of the full story of his illness and recovery. While a lofty goal, it may be possible for Ron to own his regrets without denying himself sensitive care. A fuller perspective can include regret, guilt, or shame *and* a kind sensitivity to his difficulty in facing the impact of his actions. He also has the opportunity to be proud of having the courage to accept a painful truth and make changes going forward.

Self-Talk

Self-talk can be an effective way for you to bring more sensitive understanding to your situation. The goal is to try to **coach yourself with the same warm, patient, and sensitive understanding you would give to a cherished loved one who is in a distressing situation.** Self-compassion has been shown to be effective in reducing both anger and the severity of pain. It can benefit people in chronic pain even in the absence of other pain management. It can also improve psychological well-being by decreasing anxiety, depression, and stress and increasing the capacity to accept pain.

Reminding yourself that **others can feel the same way you do** can be very valuable. We are continually surprised by how often people feel they are the only ones who feel as they do. Indeed people who recognize the universality of their feelings and their common humanity, and remember that others are also suffering, have been found to be happier, more resilient, and more satisfied with life.

To use compassionate self-talk:

- Settle into a comfortable position. You can be sitting, standing, or lying down. You might close your eyes. Open the palms of your hands and rest them on your thighs. Breathe slowly and deeply, saying the word "relax" to yourself as you exhale.

- Gently pay attention to your experience and kindly acknowledge any emotions that come up. Do your best to sensitively understand and give yourself permission to feel what you feel.

- Some find it easier to start by first bringing sensitive thoughts to someone else who is unwell or a person they love.

- Consider telling yourself:

  ○ *This is a difficult time and I am feeling agitated.*

  ○ *Living with cancer is difficult and understandably distressing.*

  ○ *It is hard to feel so unwell.*

  ○ *I feel bad that anything I did or didn't do contributed to my diagnosis.*

  ○ *I feel ashamed when I am so irritable.*

- Remind yourself of our common humanity:

  ○ *I'm not the only one who feels this way. It is normal to struggle to cope with a painful situation.*

  ○ *Coping with cancer is hard for anyone. I am only human.*

  ○ *No one is perfect.*

  ○ *Countless other people also feel irritable when they are physically or emotionally distressed.*

- When you are distracted by unkind or critical thoughts, do your best to notice the judgments and then let them pass. See if you can begin to try to understand and forgive yourself for your feelings. Ask yourself what perspectives you are missing.

  ○ *Dealing with pain and distress is hard and I am trying to learn the best ways for me to cope.*

  ○ *Some form of anger is a part of the human experience and a common response to pain*

  ○ *Even if my emotional reactions are not the same as someone else's, they make sense.*

  ○ *There is not something wrong with me.*

  ○ *What other consideration am I forgetting?*

- Learning to be kind and understanding to yourself is a gradual process. Self-compassion, like many new practices, takes time to master. Try to give yourself the same understanding you would give to a toddler who tumbles while first learning to walk. Do your best to believe you can learn to cope more effectively.

○ *It takes time to ease strong feelings, and I am still learning new tools.*

○ *The new strategies take lots of practice. They are not a one-shot cure, and everyone has to do them many times.*

• Use a warm tone that you would use with a friend, bringing warm wishes to mind as if you are asking for something or praying. Express compassion for yourself and others by internally reciting words or phrases of goodwill such as:

○ *Sorry this is so hard.*

○ *You are important and I care about you.*

○ *May I give myself the support and sensitive understanding I need.*

○ *May I learn not to be so hard on myself for my feelings and actions.*

○ *May I be healthy.*

○ *May all cancer patients be healthy.*

• Slowly repeat the phrases. Try to focus on the meaning as you say them. The mind seems able to "say" these phrases silently even when you are not paying attention to the process. See if you can focus on the meaning of the words as you gently bring your mind back to your script again and again.

• If it feels comfortable, consider giving yourself a physical gesture of kindness such as putting your hand to your heart or giving yourself a little hug.

Now we turn from your internal experience to ways to deal with your relationships to the world around you.

SEVEN

Nurturing Personal Relationships

We all have particular ways we deal with others. Are you outgoing, or is your style more reserved? Do you have a large social circle, or do you focus your time and energy on a few selectively chosen people? Perhaps you wish you had more connections. It is possible that you openly share your reactions and information with others. Maybe your style is to stay away from distressing facts or feelings or to be more private.

No matter how outgoing or private you want to be right now, and whether or not your relationships are all you want them to be, your connections to others can impact life with cancer. What's more, the way you cope may impact your relationships. This chapter offers ideas that may help nurture supportive connections. We include strategies to communicate effectively and express what you want and need.

Relationships and Cancer

Any life crisis has the potential to affect how people deal with one another. Physical, emotional, or financial challenges can influence your interactions. While some worry that cancer might strain relationships, it also has the power to deepen and enhance them.

In the face of cancer those closest to you may move even closer, while others may feel more distant. At times, a reaction feels just right. In other moments a response may surprisingly miss the mark, feeling either too coddling or too aloof. It can be hard to know how to deal with friends or family whose physical or emotional availability does not match what you need or hope for right now.

The reality is that none of us is perfect, has ideal relationships, or can change someone else. People cope and come to terms with medical information in different ways. Some folks are more idealistic or avoid painful facts, and others try to be realistic. Recall that those who tend toward emotion mind are apt to be more expressive or readily share feelings and information. Those who tend toward reasonable mind are more likely to be private and reserved. **It can be painful if a loved one's coping style does not intuitively match what works for you** at this moment.

At times people may say things intended to be helpful that unintentionally leave you feeling misunderstood. "Don't worry, I know you'll be fine" might not come across as the reassurance it's meant to be. If you experience the encouragement as minimizing what you're going through or invalidating how you're feeling, you may feel more alone. Well-intentioned suggestions such as "Use this doctor" or "Try this diet" may be useful. On the other hand, if this advice strikes you as critical of what you're doing, you may feel alienated.

If you can't be as involved with your usual sources of connection such as work, school, or physical intimacy, **you may feel isolated.** Young people can find it particularly difficult to feel cut off from the normal sense of belonging and community. Dinesh, at age 18, had days when he was too immune depressed to be in contact with anyone outside his home. He longed for everyday things that he used to take for granted like riding the subway and making small talk with fellow passengers. He described how lonely he could feel. "Some nights . . . my loneliness was convulsive. I would remind myself throughout the night of the friends whom I'd called or who had joined me at the hospital, of my parents sleeping on the floor beneath me. Still I'd struggle to fall asleep. I'd want to curl up but couldn't cuddle close enough to myself."

A need to rely on others may change the dynamic between people. Everyone responds uniquely to giving or receiving extra attention or help. Roles may change. Perhaps a family member is called on to provide additional assistance or someone who was a caregiver may now have to accept care. Some also worry about the burden or costs to their caretakers.

At this time, wittingly or unwittingly, you may be the one who is keeping a distance. Recall that when people feel vulnerable they can move into protective mode. If you believe there is a threat of not having or compromising a connection you want or need, you may put up barriers. Sometimes pulling back is a wise choice. Other times you may be reacting to inaccurate assumptions. At times protection against an unclear danger can get in the way of a closer relationship, as happened for a woman named Elena. Her hesitation to share her feelings with her husband and daughter initially compromised their relationship.

Promoting Supportive Connections

Let's follow Elena's story as an example of ways some of the skills we have already presented may help to promote supportive personal connections.

Observe

Are you telling yourself any **common relationship myths?**

- My loved ones are stressed, and it is my fault.
- I am a burden and/or needy.
- I don't deserve this time and attention.
- Asking is a sign of weakness and drives people away.
- Relationships can be harmed if one refuses to do what is asked.
- I shouldn't have to ask. My loved ones should know what I need and do it.
- I am selfish. I should give up my own needs and concerns.
- People won't want to be with me if I can't act or look like I usually do.

Try to **be aware of whether you are in emotion, reasonable, or wise mind.** Can you notice whether you're emphasizing facts or discounting your feelings and wishes as in reasonable mind? Are you jumping to conclusions, making judgmental assumptions about yourself or others in emotion mind? Do you have a wise mind perspective that balances verified facts with feelings, values, and priorities?

Elena notices how alone and needy she feels. She recognizes that some of her husband's reactions leave her feeling misunderstood. She is aware of thinking that she shouldn't share too much with her young adult daughter, believing her daughter may not be strong enough to deal with the burden and worry. Elena recognizes that she is in emotion mind.

Check the Facts

Stories we tell ourselves may feel real but are not always true. We are struck by how often people hold themselves responsible for the realities of life with cancer that are not under their control. I found managing my feelings about the impact of my cancer on my family to be one of the most challenging aspects of coping. Are you blaming yourself for a loved one's worry, stress, burden, or genetics? One man decided he wasn't the father he "wanted to be or should be" after his teenage daughter said she found visiting him at the hospital too overwhelming.

Recall the value of questioning self-critical assumptions. Can you keep in mind that you neither chose nor agreed to this reality? It is likely this situation is not your fault. Is there actually something you could have done differently to change the fact that your cancer can impact others?

Elena wonders whether she is needy. Needing someone or something means that those people or things are central to your health and happiness. It is not the same as being "needy." *Needy* is a judgment that implies there is something pitiful about you or that you aren't doing what you can to take care of yourself.

Self-Talk

When you're dealing with others, it's easy to discount your own emotions, thoughts, and right to assert yourself. Self-talk can be a valuable way to **give yourself permission to feel as you do.** In addition, when you keep in mind your connections to others, you may feel less separate and alone. Consider saying to yourself:

Many others feel as I do.

My feelings are valid even if they differ from or upset others.

I wish cancer did not also impact those around me.

I did not choose or agree to this situation.

I can try my best to accept what is out of my control.

I can't control the cards I have been dealt, but I can choose how I play them. I can decide how I want to handle my emotions and deal with others.

Relying on others is not a weakness but may be a fact of life right now.

I can appreciate all that is being done for me and need to ask for help.

Taking care of myself is not selfish and may even make it more possible for me to be able to take care of others.

There may be people who love, care about, or are praying for me who are not physically by my side at this moment.

Check the Relationship Facts

In relationships both people affect the balance of how things go, so you also want to verify your assumptions about others. Try your best to remember that you can't actually know what others are thinking unless they tell you. At times, it's useful to directly **check your assumptions with the other person.** Indeed, when asked, Elena's daughter said it was important to her to know all the details of her mother's care. Being in the loop about the information helped her feel more connected to the family and guided her decision to be more involved in her mother's care.

Listening

Listening to others is not as easy as it seems. It's challenging to adapt the story you tell yourself. Like many of us, Elena had a hard time letting go of her assumptions. She was initially convinced that it was too much for her daughter to hear about what she was going through and that a loving mother should protect her child. She had to be reminded that her daughter was an adult who had asked to know the details.

Indeed, genuinely listening requires more than just hearing another person's words. **True listening involves a willingness to try to see the world through someone else's eyes and be changed by what the person has to say.** Yet when you are unwell it can be difficult to be open to any other points of view.

The fact is that, with or without cancer, it's hard to be fully open to other perspectives. Marsha and I come from different psychological backgrounds. Writing this book together has required us to try to understand the other person's point of view without holding on to our own ideas as *the* truth. We disagreed a lot! We fought and at moments felt like it was "my way or the highway." We often had to pause and take time before realizing that perhaps the other person *was* saying something valuable. We found that we were less rigid and more willing to consider other ideas when we felt heard and respected by each other. We hung in together by keeping in mind that our priority was to try to figure out how best to help people with cancer. We like to believe that eventually listening to one another has not only brought us much closer but also made this a deeper, richer book.

Wise Mind

Wise mind, a valuable guide for making constructive decisions, can also be very useful with relationships. Do your best to consider:

- **Are you relating to others in ways that are working well for you?**

- **Are you putting your time and energy into the people who are most important to you?**

- **Do you want to change whom you focus on and/or how you relate?**

Elena recognized that her relationships with her husband and daughter meant the world to her. She decided she wanted to focus on them and not put her limited time and energy into people who were not as important to her. To consider how to strengthen her connection with them, she did her best to face the relationship facts, to be as realistic as she could about how things were going between them.

Acknowledging the truth about your relationships is not always easy. At times, it can feel as challenging as facing medical reality. Yet being realistic about your connection to those around you can help you decide whether distance makes sense in a particular relationship. Elena realized that right now she didn't feel as close to her husband and daughter as she wanted but that had not always been the case. She wondered whether it was in her interest to share more with them.

It's true that sometimes the wisest choice is not to express everything you feel. It's not always constructive to share resentment or envy. On the other hand, Elena recognized that holding back emotions does not always support a relationship. Her wise mind had helped her decide that these were reliable relationships. By choosing not to share her feelings, was she trading perceived protection for precious intimacy? Did her silence leave her daughter and husband to cope on their own? She decided it was worth her while to rethink her approach to her daughter and talk to her husband directly.

Managing Difficult Feelings

Undeniably, relationships can stir up strong emotions. Initially Elena was very annoyed by some of her husband's reactions when she talked about her cancer. She wanted to prove that her righteous indignation was justified and tried to shame, punish, and change him. Yet Elena wisely remembered that you can't actually change someone else. She realized she was wasting precious energy being unproductively angry with him and used some of the coping strategies we have presented.

Trying to minimize the intensity of her anger, Elena did her best to name her feelings and identify her thoughts and bodily reactions. She recognized her annoyance and frustration. She noticed her judgments about her husband and tried to check the facts. She used self-talk to validate her understandable irritation. In addition, she did some paced breathing to help calm her and used paired muscle relaxation and a warm, soothing bath to ease her tight muscles.

Dialectical Strategies

Elena also found it useful to keep in mind that **both people and relationships can have seemingly opposite sides that are part of the fullest picture.** She did her best to change her thinking about her daughter and their relationship. Instead of simply seeing her adult daughter as a vulnerable child, Elena tried to be open to a wider perspective about her and their relationship. She realized that, although her daughter felt fragile in some ways, Elena's diagnosis could also be, to use my sister's term, an AFGO (another frigging growth opportunity). Indeed, research shows that **in the face of crisis some people find previously untapped reservoirs of strength.**

Elena began to share more of the facts of her illness and some of her feelings with her daughter. Her faith that perhaps her daughter may be stronger than Elena initially thought gave her daughter permission to take an active role in Elena's care and allowed them to get closer. Elena and her daughter did not have to remain locked in rigid roles with the care going in only one direction. Indeed, they both became givers and receivers, supporting of *and* allowing care from one another.

A Word about Talking with Children

For many people, including me, the most difficult personal conversations about cancer are with our children. How do you honestly share what is happening in a way that a child can deal with while continuing to trust you?

Naturally, the way you talk to a child will vary with the child's age. Elena's daughter was a young adult, and the ways Elena found effective to speak with her are likely different from those you would use when talking with a younger child. On the other hand, it's easy to underestimate how much even the youngest children sense changes in their routine and are aware of the emotions and behavior of the people around them.

It's common for parents to want to protect a child by not discussing upsetting things. Yet when a child is aware of something amiss that is not being talked about, his or her imagination can sometimes be worse than the reality. Some children can get the idea that they are the cause of the distress and/or that the problem is so terrible that adults can't discuss it. Talking about these worries helps them feel less alone because they know there are people who can help them with difficult situations.

Simple honest language can eliminate confusion and misinformation. Many parents have found that using the word *cancer* helps them maintain a trusting relationship with their child. Consider saying that cancer describes cells growing more quickly than usual.

Recall that it can be easier to cope when you keep in mind the seemingly opposite ideas that a **situation can be both scary *and* hopeful.** You may want to acknowledge that the word *cancer* is scary to some people because there weren't always as many good ways to manage cancer as there are now. Share your personal treatment plan and the hope it offers. Some people describe the chemo or radiation as ways to slow down the cell growth. Over time, it's useful to explain that hair loss and other upsetting side effects are reactions to the medicine, not the illness.

As with adults, children's responses to cancer vary. Some children ask a lot of questions and want to know lots of details. Others clam up or may feel embarrassed. Some jump into caretaking, feeling they should put their lives on hold. Yet others appear to ignore what is happening, throwing themselves into their own lives. As in many other parts of life, it is most constructive to encourage a child to find a balanced middle path that also maintains his or her own life.

Questions may not come all at once, so try your best to stay open to them over time. Listen for misconceptions, such as that cancer is contagious. Some children may ask whether you're going to die. Again the goal is to balance hope and honesty. You might acknowledge the reality by saying "All of us will some day, but hopefully not from cancer" or "We hope not, and the doctors are working very hard to help me."

Other Sources of Support

Another wise mind consideration is whether sources of support outside your own intimate circle can also be helpful to you or your family at this time. Even if you have many caring and helpful people in your life, a personal and/or professional relationship with others in the community, clergy, or mental health providers may be beneficial right now.

There are many different models of cancer support. Some find it helpful to connect with people who have experience with what they are going through. One man described the value of being listened to by someone who has "been there." He said, "You don't need their words to feel understood." Cancer-specific support groups can minimize isolation, and psychosocial support has been shown to impact cancer patients' quality of life and survival rates. Other studies link social connections to pain tolerance.

Connections with others who share your experience may be available at community resources, cancer-specific settings, hospitals, or online. Some groups are specific to diagnosis, age, or stage. One woman in her 20s found friendships with others in her position by joining Breasties, a group for young people affected by breast and reproductive cancers. This particular group promotes community through social media, meetups, day events, and weekend wellness retreats. Another, more private person chose to ask her doctor to help her connect with an individual with a similar medical experience. Consider an option that suits you.

Talking Directly to Others

If you're reluctant to let others know what you want or feel you need, you're not alone. Many people hesitate to speak up. Elena was unsure how to express her concerns to her husband and also protect their relationship.

What can you do when you want to share your experience and tell someone how you really feel but the person seems to have difficulty listening? Perhaps you have a dear one who loves you so much he or she feels unable to tolerate hearing about your pain. How do you tell someone who wants to talk about what you are going through that you care about him or her but don't find talking very useful right now? Once again, we have some ideas that may help you communicate so neither of you feels bad.

Effective Communication

Direct conversation can deepen a relationship. Other people are not mind readers, and unless you speak up they don't always know what you want. Much of the time, you do need to let them know. While you can't control what others do or change them, the way you ask may influence the situation.

Constructive asking means understanding the difference between asking and demanding. When you genuinely ask, the other person has the chance to agree or not. On the other hand, a demand tells the other person what to do without giving the person the opportunity to decide whether or not to agree. Asking is respectful; a demand can damage relationships.

Keep in mind that strong emotions can impact an interaction. **It can be very valuable to use strategies to regulate your emotions before dealing with others to protect the interaction from being hindered by strong feelings.** For example, you're more likely to communicate effectively when you're less angry. It's easier to share your concerns when you're less anxious and not believing catastrophic assumptions about your relationships.

Consider looking at the skills for sadness if you're very unhappy. The sections in Chapter 6 on difficulties with self-soothing and self-talk may be valuable if you're holding yourself responsible for the way things are going with and for loved ones.

The next step is to **know your goal. What are you hoping for from the interaction?**

- Being heard and understood
- Having your view taken seriously
- Asking for a different response
- Resolving a conflict
- Getting the other person to do what you want
- Protecting a relationship
- Being liked or respected
- Maintaining or improving self-respect

Like many of us, Elena had multiple goals. Her short-term goal was to firmly ask for and get what she wanted, which was to be understood and get a different response from her husband while holding on to her long-term objective to protect their relationship.

DEAR MAN

DEAR MAN is an acronym for an effective way to ask more firmly for what you want or feel that you need:

<u>D</u>: **Describe** the situation with objective facts.

<u>E</u>: **Express** your feelings and opinions clearly.

<u>A</u>: **Assert** your wishes.

<u>R</u>: **Reinforce** the positive effects of getting what you need.

<u>M</u>: **Mindfully** pay attention to your goals and stick to them.

<u>A</u>: **Appear confident**—in tone of voice, posture, and eye contact.

<u>N</u>: **Negotiate**—be willing to give to get.

This strategy takes practice, and you may find it useful to try to plan in advance and perhaps even write out what you want to say and how you want to say it. Let's look at how Elena can use this technique to talk to her husband when their coping styles do not match. There are times she feels frightened about the future and his reaction to her anxiety leaves her feeling more alone.

Her first step is to **describe** what is bothering her. She tries to report objectively what has happened, sticking to the facts. She does her best to comment only on what she can observe—sensations, feelings, and thoughts—and **avoid making judgments and assumptions about his motives.** She says,

> *I like to turn to you when I'm upset. When I share my concerns, you often tell me everything will be fine. When I repeatedly go over the medical details, you sometimes roll your eyes.*

Next Elena tries to **express** her feelings and opinions without assuming her husband knows how she feels. Being open about your emotions can be difficult. People can be afraid of being judged, being misunderstood, or appearing weak. Honest expression means courageously sharing your feelings without a guaranteed reaction from the other person. If you are not sure the other person feels the same way as you do or will respond in kind, being vulnerable and expressing sentiments such as "I love you" may feel risky. Elena says,

> *I feel sensitive right now, and your support and approval mean a lot. Occasionally I'm upset by your reaction to me. Sometimes I believe you're trying to be encouraging, but I feel like you're just trying to placate me. When you roll your eyes, I feel like you aren't taking my concerns seriously. If I think you are critical of my coping or don't understand me, I end up feeling more alone.*

After that, she **asserts her wishes,** expressing what is helpful and what is not. She does her best to say "I want" or "I don't want" and tries to avoid saying "You should" or "You shouldn't." **If the other person expresses uncertainty about what you want, encourage the person to ask you.** Elena says,

Most of the time, I'm hoping you will simply listen. I want you to understand how scared I feel. I am often not looking to be reassured. If you don't know if it's a time for encouragement or listening, please ask me.

If the conversation is not going well, you can always express your discomfort and pause, putting the conversation off for another time. This strategy gives the other person a chance to think about your request, and you have the opportunity to ask again, perhaps in a different way. You can simply say, "Let's put this conversation on hold for now."

Elena's next step is to **reinforce** or reward her husband by telling him the positive effects of listening without automatically reassuring her. Thinking about what may be positive for the other person can mean considering the situation from his or her point of view so you have an idea of what matters. It's more effective to name the positive than the negative consequences, so try to avoid ultimatums like saying "If you don't . . . " People want to feel cared about and appreciated, so try to express gratitude where you can. Elena says,

I love you and appreciate that you are trying to be supportive and encouraging. It means so much to me to feel heard and respected. I'm more relaxed when I feel understood, and then we get along so much better.

Elena tries to stay **mindful,** which means **sticking to her point instead of getting caught in emotions.** She tries to calmly stay focused on improving communication with her husband without unwittingly compromising their relationship. She does her best not to be distracted by her own self-criticism or any comments he may be making. Like a broken record, she repeats her points in a matter-of-fact way.

Your support is so important to me. I really hope you can listen to me and understand that I am scared without reassuring or judging me.

Elena strives to **appear confident** and approach the conversation optimistic that it will go well. She makes an effort to use a strong tone of voice, without stammering or whispering. She tries to appear self-assured in her physical manner and posture, looking him in the eye instead of staring at the floor.

Finally, Elena is willing to **negotiate,** which means being willing to give to get. She is open to finding other ways to improve the situation. She tries to focus on what will work and asks her husband for ideas on how they can solve the problem.

GIVE

GIVE is an acronym for a strategy that helps to **maintain or strengthen an important relationship** by asking for something in a way that still allows you and the other person to feel good about and respect each other.

<u>G</u>: **Gentle:** Be nice and respectful

<u>I</u>: **Interested:** Appear interested in what the other person has to say

<u>V</u>: **Validate:** Show your understanding of the other person

<u>E</u>: **Easy manner:** Be lighthearted, smile, and consider using humor

This approach can help Elena balance her immediate objective of having her husband respond to her in a different way with her long-term goal of protecting their relationship. Let's look at how she can use this tool so she and her husband can maintain a sense of being on the same team instead of fighting one another. As Elena is initially irritated at him, she uses paced breathing and paired muscle relaxation to calm herself before she begins to talk.

She focuses on using a **gentle** manner for the conversation, trying to avoid attacks, threats, judging, and disrespect or guilt trips. Instead of suggesting it is "my way or the highway" or making the issue her husband's problem, she proposes they **share responsibility for improving what is happening between them.**

This is such a hard time for both of us. Perhaps we are both upset with the situation and not supporting each other in the best way. Can we both see if we can find a way to work together to improve our communication?

She tries to act **interested** in his perspective about the situation by facing him, leaning in, and maintaining eye contact without interrupting him. She assumes he is annoyed and critical of her rehashing medical information but gently checks it out with him.

I like to talk about the facts and my feelings. I appreciate that you have your own reactions to my cancer, and I want to try to also understand your perspective. What is it like for you when I talk about how upset I am and keep reviewing the medical facts?

Her husband was not initially open to the conversation, and Elena wisely was sensitive to his wish to talk about their troubles at another time. He felt respected by her and was much more open the second time around. If you are not making progress with repeated conversations, consider reaching out to a mental health professional, member of the clergy, or other supportive person to help you talk to one another.

Validating her husband was crucial to their successful conversation. Even though she remained clear that she did not agree with how he was communicating, Elena made sure to do and say things to let her husband know that his feelings, thoughts, and actions were understandable to her.

Maybe our communication is strained because we have different ways of coping. I like to review the details with others and share my feelings. It seems like you prefer to be more private and less emotional. Is there a way we can be more sensitive and respectful of each other's style?

Finally, Elena uses an **easy manner,** remembering that you "catch more flies with honey than with vinegar." She smiles and uses a light manner, sweet-talking him for a soft sell.

GIVE allowed them to agree that he will try to ask for and be open to feedback on how his reactions are coming across to her and she will try to speak up gently when she is feeling misunderstood.

A Word about Physical Intimacy

Communication about the physical and emotional aspects of intimate relationships may seem challenging right now. At times people may worry that changes in traditional physical intimacy will compromise the whole relationship. Try to notice whether you are "catastrophizing" in emotion mind. Do your best to pay attention to whether you're keeping a distance from your partner to protect yourself from feeling vulnerable or if your partner is feeling pushed away by the distance. You want to be sure that your reluctance to share your concerns is not compromising your emotional intimacy. At times, it can be difficult but extremely valuable to say "I don't feel desirable right now, but I still love you and want you to love me." The book *Sex and Cancer*, listed in the Notes, may also be helpful at this time.

Try to keep in mind the value of gentle touch, back rubs and other forms of massage, hand-holding, kissing, or caressing. Recall that a 20-second hug along with 10 minutes of hand-holding can be an invaluable source of comfort and affection, lowering your response to stress and anxiety.

Next we turn to relationships in your larger world, with medical providers and colleagues.

EIGHT

Communicating with Colleagues and Medical Professionals

Cancer can have an impact on how you relate to people inside and outside your intimate circle. If you're hesitant to let people in your larger world know what you want or to voice your concerns, you are not alone.

It can be difficult to know how to effectively discuss your ongoing paid or volunteer involvement in your community or workplace. Are you trying to figure out how much information you want to share? It can also be challenging to navigate the medical world with major decisions to be made and complicated finances to negotiate. Do you have as much explanation as you need to digest complex information that can have significant physical, emotional, and financial implications? Are you wishing for more time and/or other opinions to understand your situation more fully?

Sometimes emotions can get in the way of effectively asking for what you hope for. At times you may blame yourself or those around you for difficulty negotiating a complex medical world. Perhaps you worry about being too demanding, or that your anger will alienate someone you need to depend on right now. Is pride getting in the way of speaking up? Do you feel frustrated, overwhelmed, or intimidated? Are you tempted to give up trying to get time, information, and resources that may be in your interest?

As difficult as it may seem, there are **effective ways to ask for the sensitivity, information, and assistance or respect that is important to you *and* protect relationships that may be central to your well-being.** In this chapter we show you how to apply the strategies presented so far for making decisions, managing emotions, and promoting supportive relationships to help you talk with colleagues and medical professionals. We introduce the skill FAST, a way to express your wishes without compromising how you feel about yourself.

Your Relationship with Your Medical Provider

At this time there may be more dimensions to your connection with your doctor than you realize. On one hand, you are a consumer looking for vital medical expertise. Yet dealing with high-stakes medical concerns can touch core personal issues. Right now your doctor may feel as central to your existence as your ties to your nearest and dearest. Perhaps you are also hoping to be sensitively understood. Indeed, a supportive relationship with a physician has been shown to significantly impact a patient's emotional state.

Most physicians are sensitive and kind. Yet a doctor often has limited time, and your time with your doctor may be briefer than you wish. At times a well-intentioned comment may miss the mark for you. "We will get to that" or "Don't worry" may come across as unresponsive or indifferent. Have you ever felt things that troubled you were not being taken seriously? Sometimes people feel the complexity of their experience is inadvertently trivialized. At other moments some may feel misunderstood and/or judged.

Consider Tyrone's story:

I was lying down curled up in a ball when my doctor came in to examine me. He appeared to be annoyed and said, "Sit up; you're not dying!"

Feeling like a belittled child, I tried to gather my confidence to say what was on my mind. Although I was too intimidated to request anything, I thought I was not supposed to consult anyone else. I hesitantly asked whether my doctor would explain a different treatment option. Am I a candidate? Can I talk to another patient who has been through that procedure?

I watched his face like a hawk. Did he only seem to twitch? He seemed bored, and I imagined he thought I was wasting his time. He probably just wanted to get back to his research. Did he avoid looking me in the eye because my prognosis was so poor? I felt judged and demeaned when he said, "I see you are the nervous type, so we can do the scan earlier." Was he implying there was something wrong with me for being so nervous and requiring so much explanation?

The whole exam left me reeling. I felt more like a piece of machinery being lubricated or trimmed than a real person who might feel vulnerable and have feelings. Should I just change doctors, or he is a competent physician and I am just expecting too much?

How can you most constructively address concerns like Tyrone's?

Observe

Once again, the key is to be as clear as possible about the facts of the situation as well as your own heart and mind. Recall the importance of distinguishing things that actually happened from assumptions and judgments. Tyrone tries to identify the objective information he can detect from his senses. He is aware that his heart is pounding. He names his emotions: agitation, annoyance, and anxiety. He recognizes the facts are that he was lying down when the doctor came in. Tyrone questioned him. He closely watched the doctor and had theories about what he saw.

As many of us do, Tyrone realized he had assumptions and judgments about himself and his doctor. His ideas included **common myths about physicians**:

- Medical doctors are not concerned with feelings.
- Questions annoy and waste the doctor's time.
- You may not be told the truth.
- A second opinion is disloyal and can compromise the relationship.
- Doctors do not welcome patient input and may not respect their decision making.
- If you speak up, you will be labeled as a DP—difficult patient.

The balance between Tyrone's feelings, personal preferences, and quality-of-life concerns is askew. He feels a strong urge to act on his emotions and recognizes that he is in emotion mind.

Check the Facts

Checking the facts is crucial. Sometimes an assumption about your doctor may be accurate. Other times your ideas may not be.

The common stereotype is that medical doctors discount feelings, possibly their own as well as yours. They are often pigeonholed in reasonable mind. Indeed, reasonable-mind physicians, pressed for time, may prioritize medical expertise over emotions, personal preferences, or quality-of-life considerations. They are sometimes judged as insensitive. One woman tells the story of a doctor who sent her for a psychiatric evaluation after she took extra time to consult other medical professionals, family members, financial advisers, and clergy before making a difficult treatment decision.

Yet all doctors are not the same. While the reasonable-mind stereotype may apply to some physicians, many physicians are often in wise mind. They try their best to balance medical expertise *and* sensitive respect for your concerns. They believe that a vital part of their job is helping you understand your situation so you can make the best decisions for yourself. They can be very supportive of a second opinion and do not view it as a personal affront to their competence.

Dialectical Strategies

Right now it's hard for Tyrone to consider anything other than his own perspective. Yet there are always other ways to look at a situation. Can he do his best to say "Wait a minute—what else should I be considering?" Pausing to take that helicopter view can help him expand his narrow outlook to take into account another viewpoint that could also be true.

Could his doctor's comment "You're not dying" have been intended to be encouraging and reassuring? Is it possible that what came across as an irritated tone was not the doctor's reaction to Tyrone's lying down but to something unrelated to Tyrone? He reminds himself that neither he nor his doctor is a mind reader. They can observe each other's actions. Yet they can't know how the other is responding because you can't know what someone else is thinking or feeling. Perhaps "I see you are the nervous type" was an attempt to be empathic. Is Tyrone's rapid heartbeat a reaction to the doctor's communication style? Could it also be from Tyrone's anxiety about his medical status? Tyrone imagines his doctor is not being candid about his poor prognosis. Has Tyrone been clear about how much honest information he wants to hear? Could his doctor be trying to protect him as physicians trying to be sensitive can sometimes do? Perhaps the prognosis is not as poor as Tyrone fears.

Self-Talk

It is valuable for Tyrone to consider other perspectives without discounting his own experience. He also tries to give himself permission to feel as he does and validate his right to ask for what is important to him.

> *I am living with cancer. This is a difficult time. It is natural that I may feel more emotional and vulnerable right now.*
>
> *I am being too hard on myself. My thoughts and feelings make sense in this situation.*
>
> *It is reasonable to be self-respecting and ask for what is important to me.*
>
> *I can both appreciate my doctor's expertise and hope for more time, information, or responsiveness.*
>
> *Most people want to be sensitively understood.*

Face the Facts

At times it can be extremely hard to accept painful realities. When we're unwell, we want to believe our doctors are infallible because we rely on them for our health. It's understandable that we want to be confident that they have all the answers and effective remedies we need. We count on them to give us the tests and treatments that will cure us faster. We want to see them as medical wizards who know prognostic statistics so they must know what the future holds for us.

It can be extremely challenging to face the fact that our doctors are anything other than the perfect gods we (or they) wish they could be for us. We don't want to acknowledge that the limits of modern medicine may restrict their ability to help us. We don't want to see that they might be having an off moment or their own difficulties addressing painful realities. Facing that they can be as human as the rest of us may mean accepting that no mortal has all the answers we want. Not an easy task!

If his doctor is not perfect, does Tyrone have to give up hope of being helped? Can he keep in mind that things are not one way or the other?

There may be a middle ground, where doctors are neither infallible *nor* unable to help. Keeping the fullest perspective in mind may help Tyrone have both a realistic view of his doctor *and* remain hopeful.

Wise Mind

Tyrone looks to his wise mind to focus on what is most important to him. He wants to be as clear as he can about his priorities in this relationship. He knows that a physician's expertise and responsiveness to his medical needs are vital. Is his doctor's emotional sensitivity also crucial to him? Is it important for his doctor to hear, understand, and respect what is important to him?

Tyrone also considers how much involvement he wants in treatment decisions. Does he want to be reassured by a clear recommendation without going into too much detail? Perhaps it matters to him to have all possible options and their implications laid out for him. Are there things Tyrone is hoping to discuss with his doctor? Is it important to him to feel he has some part in making decisions and/or to have his input respected? He considers whether he wants to express his wishes about the way he hopes things will go if the end seems near. Is there truly a risk that raising issues could compromise a relationship with someone so vital to his care? Does his self-respect depend on speaking up nonetheless?

Tyrone's wise mind recognizes that he respects his doctor's medical expertise and is pleased with his physical care. Yet he does not feel he is getting the emotional responsiveness he hopes for. Does he have to trade one for the other? He is aware that it is important to him to have a relationship that balances medical expertise *and* sensitive understanding and so tries to make a decision that reflects those values.

Tyrone doesn't want his emotions to drive an impulsive choice to simply switch to a doctor he thinks will listen more carefully. Nor does he want to settle for just going along with a distressing situation. He considers options others have found helpful.

- **Cope ahead** by writing out in advance questions and issues to be discussed, including how much honest information he wants to hear and/or input he wants to give.

- **Use emotion regulation strategies before talking to the doctor** to minimize the risk that emotions will get in the way of effective communication.

- **Take notes or record the meeting** so he can review and ask for further explanation at a later time.

- **Take along another person (family, friend, advocate, or patient navigator)** to take notes and help ask questions.

- **Raise questions with a different person who has more time** to address the concerns—perhaps either someone else in the doctor's office (nurse or physician's assistant) or a second opinion.

- **Talk with another patient** who has had a similar procedure.

- **Use emotion regulation skills** after the meeting to manage difficult feelings.

Effective Communication

If Tyrone decides to have a direct talk with his doctor, the skills presented in Chapter 7 may help him express his concerns and hopes while also maintaining self-respect and a constructive working relationship. Tyrone's doctor can't know that it is important to Tyrone to have his options explained sensitively and have some input in decisions unless Tyrone speaks up. He considers what he hopes to get from talking with his doctor. He has a number of goals. He wants to be heard and understood, get a different response so he feels his concerns are taken seriously, protect his relationship with the doctor, yet maintain his self-respect.

Tyrone recalls that **DEAR MAN helps us ask firmly** and **GIVE helps us maintain and strengthen a relationship.** He can also consider using the skill **FAST** to help him **maintain and strengthen self-respect.**

FAST

FAST can be a useful strategy for communicating with professionals in a way that also respects your own values and beliefs. People sometimes overapologize for making valid requests. Unnecessary apologies can undermine credibility and self-confidence. This approach can help you feel capable and effective after the interaction, whether or not you get the results or changes you want:

F: Be **fair** to yourself and the other person—validating both of your feelings and wishes.

A: **Assert** wishes and priorities **without apologizing** for making a request, having an opinion or disagreeing.

S: **Stick to your own values**—be clear about what you value as a moral way of thinking.

T: Be **truthful**—don't exaggerate or make up excuses, lie, or act helpless when you are not.

Tyrone wonders whether his desires are unreasonable or he is being too needy. He does some research and recognizes that he has gotten all the information he can on his own. After considering his deepest values, he decides to ask for more time from his doctor to raise his treatment concerns because it is so important to him and his family.

Let's look at how Tyrone might integrate DEAR MAN, GIVE, and FAST to talk with his doctor. Using the DEAR MAN framework, he might start by **describing** his situation, trying to avoid judgments and assumptions about his doctor's motives. He tries to use an easy manner, being gentle and respectful of both himself and his doctor. He does his best to be fair and not exaggerate the problem.

I had some questions and things I wanted to discuss at our last appointment. I left feeling upset.

He **expresses** his feelings and opinions without assuming his physician knows how he felt. Although it's hard, Tyrone attempts to be as clear as he can about his own experience in the interaction. Openly expressing concerns can sometimes improve a relationship and deepen the other person's compassion.

I felt intimidated and believed you disapproved of my being so anxious. I thought my questions were annoying and wasting your time but that you would be upset if I asked anyone else. I also worried you didn't think I could handle bad news and so were not telling me everything.

He **asserts** his wishes and priorities without apologizing for his feelings.

I want to know as much honest information as I can even if it is bad news. I am hoping for sensitivity and respect about how I feel and what is important to me.

Tyrone **reinforces** the positive effects of getting what he needs. He keeps FAST in mind and sticks to what is important to him.

I am calmer when I assume I am understood and accepted. When so much in my life feels out of my control, it helps me to know as much information as I can and have input on the decisions.

Tyrone attempts to be **mindful** of his goal of improving his working relationship with his doctor while maintaining his self-respect. He tries to balance asserting a valid message with exaggerating the problem. He attempts to show some understanding of the doctor and not put him on the defensive. He does his best to be fair and truthful. He assumes his doctor's intentions are positive unless proven otherwise.

I realize you might have been trying to encourage me or protect me, or perhaps you appeared irritated about things that don't involve me.

He attempts to **appear confident**. He tries to avoid appearing ashamed by pulling his shoulders back and keeping his head up. He does his best to make good eye contact and use a strong voice without apologizing for his feelings.

He **negotiates** in an effort to encourage his doctor to also be open to making changes. He tries to show some willingness to take responsibility for how the relationship is going.

I know we are both doing our best in a difficult situation. I am trying to find ways to manage my emotions, including noticing my assumptions. I am trying to remember not to jump to conclusions and consider other possibilities before reacting. If you are pressed for time, is there someone else you work with who would have more time to talk with me?

Relationships with Colleagues

At times, cancer may also affect how you relate to those you work with in the community or workplace. Are you questioning how much medical or personal information you want to share? Are you wondering whether your relationship will change if you're open about your current status? Perhaps you're trying to figure out how to balance allowing or requesting help without feeling you will be discounted, pitied, or feel like a burden. If you decide to talk with others, what do you say?

Tyrone feels vulnerable and isolated and is unsure about how he wants to connect to people in his office.

> *Do I have to tell people at work what is going on with me? I'm private, and people gossip. My colleagues will treat me differently. They'll keep their distance and stop turning to me. I hate the idea of being seen as weak or being pitied.*
>
> *Still, I'm tired, and it's harder to focus. My memory isn't as sharp as usual. What is the matter with me? My friend didn't seem to have problems working. Someone suggested I look into disability insurance. I'm not disabled. I would have to share personal information to apply. Is my pride getting in the way of getting support? I don't want to jeopardize my health insurance or job. I'd better keep quiet and tough it out.*

Let's look at how the strategies for making decisions, managing emotions, and promoting supportive relationships may help you or Tyrone decide how to communicate effectively with colleagues.

Observe

What objective information can Tyrone detect from his senses? His energy is low, and he feels lethargic. His brain seems foggy, and his chest is heavy and hollow. He has butterflies in his stomach, and he feels as if he is a tight bundle of nerves.

He names his emotions. He is frightened, anxious, angry, and sad. Can Tyrone recognize that he is in emotion mind, where it's hard to remember that you can't know the future or what others are feeling or thinking?

He tries to pay attention to the difference between facts and assumptions. The reality right now is that Tyrone's current status is making it harder to work in the same way as usual. He feels distant from his colleagues. He does his best to recognize his judgments. His view of himself changes as he imagines that his cancer now defines him. He compares himself to his friend and decides he must be weak. He worries that his current difficulties are permanent. He decides he will be irrelevant to his coworkers if he can't contribute in the same ways.

He makes assumptions about the future that include **common myths about colleagues:**

My coworkers won't be sensitive and understanding.

My privacy won't be respected. Others expect to know my medical status and then won't keep the information confidential.

People will keep their distance.

They will stare at my changed appearance but not talk to me. Rumors will go around about what is wrong with me.

I will be a burden.

Coworkers will discount me, thinking I am not up to the task or that I'm leaving or dying.

Check the Facts

Once again, it's important to know that your thoughts are trustworthy. Sometimes your beliefs are correct, and other times they are not. Accurate information informs wise decisions.

Talking with his doctor about the ways health impacts his work can help Tyrone get a reliable and realistic perspective of his situation. Is he comparing himself to idealized images of strong cancer patients that overly simplify life with cancer? Mild cognitive changes sometimes referred to as "chemo brain" are common and usually subside. Tyrone assumes his office will be unresponsive to his needs. He makes broad generalizations, presuming all his coworkers will be insensitive and not respect his confidentiality. He is especially worried because a coworker's medical situation is freely discussed in the office. Is this fact a reliable indicator of how his situation will be handled? Does he have confirmed information about the nature and culture of his office or the availability of short- or long-term disability insurance?

Dialectical Strategies

Tyrone tries to remember that there are many possible ways to look at a situation. Can he do his best to take a broader, more balanced perspective?

At times there is more to a story than we realize. Just as Tyrone's story may or may not apply to you, generalizations from another's situation are not always applicable. Tyrone's assumptions about confidentiality in his office do not take the whole story into consideration. His ideas leave out information particular to his colleague's case. Unlike Tyrone, this coworker has been clear that she is comfortable with shared information and does not feel her privacy is disregarded.

Tyrone considers whether it's possible that some individuals in his office will respond sensitively. The full story may not be as simple as all his colleagues keeping their distance. Sometimes a coworker doesn't reach out because he or she is uncomfortable, doesn't know how to deal with the situation, or is trying to respect your privacy. When people don't want to say or do the wrong thing, they sometimes do nothing at all. Is it possible that there are respectful coworkers who care very much and value Tyrone's contribution? They may be very eager to hear how they can be most supportive of him.

Face the Facts

On the other hand, there are times when the truth is painful. Checking the facts and using dialectical strategies do not automatically guarantee an optimistic picture. As difficult as it may be, doing your best to face the reality is crucial to making wise decisions.

It's not easy for Tyrone to acknowledge that right now he's having trouble working the same way as in the past. He is very tired and is having trouble concentrating. His insurance and income are important to his family. He also has to accept the difficult reality that, cancer or no cancer, no one can definitively answer his questions about the future. Despite valuable input from his doctor, Tyrone may have to tolerate some uncertainty about his work life going forward.

Self-Talk

It's very valuable to be kind to yourself. Try your best to remind yourself:

It's not uncommon for cancer to affect people's capacity to engage in activities in their usual way.

Changes in how I'm working right now are not necessarily permanent.

Any limitations are likely not the result of something I did or didn't do.

There is more to me than doing things as I always have in the past. Working in a different way doesn't have to define my relationships or me.

Dealing with cancer is not easy for anyone even though someone else's struggles may not be obvious.

I'm learning new ways to handle these challenges even though they take practice. These ideal steps are easier said than done.

Wise Mind

Tyrone can make the most effective decisions about communicating with his colleagues when he balances the facts with his own heart and mind. He tries his best to consider information and input from others without losing sight of what is most important to him. Ultimately he is the best judge of how he feels physically and emotionally and what is most beneficial for him at this time.

As happens for many, Tyrone's cancer threatens his already delicate work/life balance. He now has even more priorities to juggle. In addition to everything else, it is now especially important for him to take care of his physical and emotional health while protecting his job and health benefits. At the same time, he wants to maintain his privacy and self-respect. Tyrone looks to his wise mind to ensure he is constructively balancing his priorities to make trade-offs that are in his interest.

His first instinct is not to tell anyone that he is having trouble working the same way as usual. He considers the pros and cons of sharing this information. Tyrone's work is an important source of income and a useful distraction at this time. He doesn't want to open a discussion about whether or not he is capable of working right now. He assumes if he lets people know what he's going through they will gossip, judge, and/or ostracize him. He worries that having people know his current situation could harm his job security. If his assumptions are accurate, he may be wise to keep quiet.

On the other hand, a wise mind also considers the cost of silence. Marsha has personally found that telling people she has trouble with her memory and asking for help has not affected how much they like her. On the other hand she thinks that denying the problem may get in the way of a relationship or a job. Tyrone also questions whether his job is in more jeopardy if his coworkers don't understand why he is not working as usual. He wonders whether there are laws that protect him. Does being so private increase his isolation and leave him feeling lonelier?

In addition, Tyrone is concerned about his self-respect. Understandably, economic insecurity can shake one's sense of control. It's important to him to feel he contributes and makes a difference to others. Is he less likely to judge himself as weak or a burden if he tries to "tough it out" without telling people what he's going through? Others find that working at this time is a terrible burden and may be upset that colleagues are expecting too much of them. Their focus right now may be on putting their time and energy into their health and family. Is there a self-respecting way to express whatever your concerns are?

In wise mind, Tyrone tries to take a balanced perspective, remembering that things are not one way *or* the other. He is not strong *or* weak. Inability to do everything in the way he did in the past does not define him as useless. Tyrone recognizes that his income, health benefits, connection with colleagues, and self-respect are important to him right now. He wants to work as much as possible.

Perhaps there is also a middle path to communicating with his colleagues. Is it possible to choose to confide only in reliable individuals who are nonjudgmental and will respect his confidentiality? If he can speak in a way that protects his dignity, he decides that selectively sharing his current status with sensitive and supportive people is a worthwhile trade-off.

In deciding what might be helpful, he considers **ways others have dealt with attention or memory difficulties, fatigue, and the wish to stay involved.** Some of the most useful ideas include:

- Minimizing distractions
  - Working in a setting that is as enclosed as possible, like a room with a door that closes
  - Working in quieter areas or using earplugs
- Keeping to-do lists and strategically placed sticky notes
- Limiting multitasking by completing one task at a time
- Taking frequent work breaks
- Having flex hours
- Working from home
- Working on discrete projects
- Having a trusted coworker offer a second set of eyes
- Referring to *cancerandcareers.org* or *askjan.org* (job accommodation network)

Emotion Regulation

Tyrone also recognizes that he can communicate more effectively if he is less anxious, sad, angry, or critical of himself. He reviews the strategies presented earlier for minimizing intense emotion and self-talk. He **chooses which skills will be in his interest to use before he speaks.**

Talking to Colleagues

Let's look at how Tyrone can use the communication strategies we have presented to let a colleague know what he is going through so he can feel less alone and more understood. His goal is to clearly express what might be helpful to him at this time.

Once again he uses the DEAR MAN framework to ask for what he wants and keeps GIVE and FAST in mind to protect his relationships and self-respect.

He begins by **describing** his situation. Sharing his circumstances educates his coworkers about a common problem with cancer and helps him feel less alone.

I have been reluctant to share that I have cancer and some difficulty concentrating, which can be a common short-term side effect.

He **expresses** his feelings and opinions. It can be especially hard to share vulnerability in a work setting, yet doing so sometimes deepens a relationship and another's compassion.

It is hard to feel that parts of my life are out of my control. I am still trying to figure out places I can influence things. It is helpful to feel I can have some control over my privacy and dignity.

He **asserts** his wishes and priorities.

I'd like to feel that my wish for privacy could be respected and that I have some influence over what is shared about me. Please don't feel a need to say anything special to make me feel better or reassure me. I only hope to know that my work and life make a difference to others. It would mean a lot if people would continue to turn to me to contribute.

He **reinforces** the positive aspects of getting what he is asking for.

It's very helpful to me to feel competent and stay engaged in the parts of my life that are not about cancer. Feeling that my input is valued and my privacy is respected is very important to me. I found it particularly supportive when one person commented on my weight loss by saying he wanted to respect my privacy but also have me know he cared about me.

Tyrone tries to stay **mindful** of his goal of keeping a good working relationship with his colleague while maintaining his self-respect. He keeps GIVE and FAST in mind, attempting to use an easy, light manner, while trying to be sensitive to his own concerns as well as the other person's.

I recognize that people have their own reactions to hearing this news and that some may wish to talk to others or share the news out of concern for me. I appreciate the caring interest but want to minimize the conversation.

He does his best to **appear confident,** using a strong voice and making eye contact. He pulls his shoulders back and keeps his head up.

Tyrone also tries to **negotiate,** showing his willingness to "give to get."

If you have concerns about my health or work or are unsure whether I want to talk about my situation, please ask me directly. I will try to be open about things that impact work and be clear if there are times I would rather not discuss other issues.

In the next and final chapter, we go into more depth on living in a way that is consistent with what matters most to you.

NINE

Living Meaningfully

After a cancer diagnosis, some people reassess their priorities and consider how they want to live now. Physical, emotional, and/or financial comfort and security may be more important at this time. Issues of faith and spirituality may seem more central. Some may feel more alone or disconnected from who or what usually carries and guides them. They may wonder how to have hope and trust in an unpredictable world or question whether their life has been or can continue to be meaningful.

Many find this to be a valuable opportunity to deepen their connection to what matters most. They may devote more time and energy to the people, activities, values, ideals, and beliefs that are most significant to them. Living meaningfully can seem challenging even when you don't have cancer, yet it is always possible to have or build a meaningful life.

Indeed, it may be worth your while to try. Many discover that reaffirming who or what is important to them and/or choosing to live more in tune with their priorities builds confidence and improves their relationships and the way they live. Research has shown that people with advanced cancer who focused their energy on what was most meaningful to them felt less hopeless and depressed.

In this final chapter we review the ways some of the key skills we have presented may help you connect to what is meaningful to you. We also introduce two more strategies, **half-smiling** and **willing hands.**

Face the Facts

The first step to making any changes is to honestly pay attention to the reality of your life right now. Marsha uses the term **radical acceptance** to describe the process of realistically acknowledging those challenging moments that occur in our lives. The difficulties can range from day-to-day frustrations to inevitable bodily changes over your life span to cancer's impact on your life.

Facing the facts can be challenging. We wish certain realities weren't the case. Naturally, we dislike any limitations on our ability to do things that are important to us. We certainly don't want any negative impacts on our family. It may be hard to keep in mind that admitting the truth does not mean we agree with what is happening. At times, we think we would be happier if we ignored certain facts. Even Marsha, a Zen master who spent years teaching people about radical acceptance, recently noticed her initial reluctance to hear how much pain was entailed in a surgery for a condition much less serious than cancer.

We may believe that we don't have the courage to look an upsetting or scary reality in the eye. We may worry about being overwhelmed by our feelings or giving up if we admit how serious things are. We may forget that it is possible to face the facts *and* still work toward change and that there are effective ways to handle strong feelings.

Life with cancer can seem radically difficult to face. In the normal course of events, our world may appear relatively predictable and we may feel more or less in control. We typically assume our questions can be answered definitively and don't spend time thinking about unknowns. Day-to-day life doesn't usually require us to focus on the fact that we can't know what the future holds and that we will all die some day. Yet cancer may stir up these issues. Now we may be suddenly confronted with the uncertainties of life and the limits of our control. We may be forced to recognize our mortality. We may be disappointed, angry, or doubtful. We can have many questions: "Am I going to be okay?" "How did this happen?" "Do bad things really happen to good people?" "Why me?" Faced with so many unknowns, it can be hard to accept that it may not be possible to get the definitive answers we want.

It can be traumatic to realistically see the limits of our control and/ or acknowledge the ultimate uncertainty of how long we will live. Intense emotions may be stirred. An ordinarily quite confident man named Thomas described feeling trapped and full of self-doubt. Referencing the song *My Ride's Here*, written by Warren Zevon after Zevon was diagnosed with a terminal illness, Thomas now questioned whether he had pursued his highest goals and lived fully. Had he wasted his life because he hadn't yet read all the great books? Had he been a good enough father and husband?

So why on earth do we suggest it might be useful to try to acknowledge the fact that you can't know how long you will live? Accepting the realities of what we are unable to control can help us make more effective decisions. In a threatening situation our first coping instincts aren't always the most productive. Consider the urge to run from a bear or slam on the brakes when your car is skidding on the ice. The more productive responses are actually the opposite. Don't run and gently pump your brakes, respectively.

Similarly, an inclination to be self-critical, avoid a difficult treatment, or back off from people and activities that are supportive and nourishing may not be the most effective approach. Looking at the full story, including the drawbacks of an initial reaction, may motivate more constructive choices. Maybe you start to take better care of yourself and/or follow medical advice. Indeed, when Marsha accepted the medical necessity of the surgery she initially wanted to avoid, she went ahead with it.

Coming to terms with an uncertain future and facing the fact that we all die sometime may help you deepen your connection to who or what is most significant to you. **Many find that acknowledging a risk of losing precious time and relationships helps them treasure life right now, live more in tune with their values, and cherish the people they really care about.** Thomas started to put more time into family dinners and trips and spend one-on-one time with loved ones to maximize those connections. He also began to reengage his creative talents, prioritizing work on social issues.

What's more, trying to maintain control may be unrealistic and get in the way of enjoying life as fully as possible. Certain activities require us to let go so we can experience their full pleasure. Consider what may happen with skiing, sailing, riding a bike, or surfing. In these activities, we may need to accept the futility of holding on to the illusion of total control in order to be willing to allow our skis to face downhill, let out our sail in the wind, ride the wave, or take off on that bicycle. In the same way, we may miss the full joy of being somewhere or with someone if we are only half there because we are so focused on trying to control what is happening. Facing your mortality can feel like the ultimate letting go. On the other hand, accepting this truth about life can be a **powerful incentive to think more about how you want to live while you are still alive.** You may be motivated to take the seemingly counterintuitive step of **living as fully and meaningfully as you can for as long as you can.**

How to Face Distressing Facts

We do recognize that "Easier said than done" may not come close to capturing the difficulty of accepting that you may not be living the way you want or the ultimate uncertainty about whether you will live as long as you hoped or planned. Still, it is possible that even if you doubt yourself or feel very vulnerable right now, you may also be more capable of coping than you ever imagined. Do your very best to keep in mind that **it's possible to *both* feel very overwhelmed *and* be wiser, stronger, and more courageous than you think.** You have reason to have faith in your ability to cope because you may already have more skills in your toolbox than you realize. Many of the same strategies we have presented for coping when life is unpredictable and throws you off balance may now be helpful in facing distressing events. Let's review the steps that can be used again and again as you try to come to terms with upsetting truths.

Mindfulness

As you consider what you have to face, do your very best to keep in mind that **your voice and heart always matter.** Try to pay attention to your physical sensations, thoughts, and emotions and how they impact each other. Recall the value of the open-palm image, doing your best to allow these sensations, ideas, and feelings to come, notice them, and then let them go.

Physical Sensations

Can you notice your bodily sensations? Consider using **paced breathing** and/or **paired muscle relaxation,** presented in Chapter 3, to impact your body to regulate your emotion. Two additional strategies may be helpful in facing difficult facts.

Willing hands can send a message from your hands to your brain to be more open to considering a difficult reality.

- Drop your arms down from your shoulders. If you're standing, keep them straight or bent slightly at the elbows. If you're sitting, place them on your lap or thighs. If you're lying down, leave them at your side.
- Turn your hands outward, with your hands unclenched, thumbs out to your sides, palms up, and fingers relaxed.

Half-smiling may help communicate a more accepting stance to your brain while considering a difficult reality.

- Relax your face from the top of your head down to your chin and jaw. Let go of each facial muscle (forehead, eyes, brows, cheeks, mouth, and tongue). Allow your teeth to be slightly apart. If you're having difficulty, try to tense your facial muscles and then let go. A tense smile is a grin that might tell your brain you are hiding or masking real feelings.
- Let both corners of your lips go slightly up, just so you can feel them. It is not necessary for others to see it. A half smile is slightly upturned lips with a relaxed face.
- Try to adopt a serene facial expression.

Thoughts

Do you notice a reluctance to be realistic about your situation? Is there a shift in your faith in yourself, your relationships, or the larger world? Are you aware of thinking more about the future than how you are living at present?

Cancer is hard enough without adding self-judgment. Watch out for assumptions about yourself, your current abilities, and your relationships. Beware of unconstructive ideas such as that your life is meaningless or that you can't still make a difference to others and no longer have a place.

Notice if you're criticizing yourself because, like many of us, your actions are not always consistent with your priorities. Try to be sensitive to how difficult it is to accept painful realities or focus on anything other than your health concerns right now. Feeling too preoccupied with fears about the future to pay attention to living meaningfully is understandable.

Keep in mind that it may be valuable to **check the facts** to assess your assumptions about yourself and your dear ones. Your ideas about what you realistically do have to accept may not be accurate. Your worst fears may not always come true. Some people regain capacities and/or live longer than they or their doctor ever expected. Since you can't ever definitively know the future, it may be very helpful to check out your assumptions with your doctor, family, and your own wise mind. Do your best to **keep in mind that there is always reason for hope.**

Can you notice whether you're in emotion or reasonable mind? See if you can take a more **balanced wise mind** view, remembering that things are not necessarily one way *or* the other. Your current situation may not be as simple as still doing everything in the same way *or* being unable to live a meaningful life. Most likely your life is neither perfect nor meaningless. None of us lives an ideal life in tune with all our values or has relationships that are all we want them to be. It's very hard to do all the things we want to do. All of us have done things we wish we hadn't done. Most of us haven't lived in ways we promised ourselves we would live. Those who need to say they're sorry have the opportunity to do so. The truth is that even if you can't do everything you used to do or your relationships are not ideal, you're not helpless. You have a choice about how you play the cards you are dealt.

Consider using **self-talk** to give yourself the understanding and compassion you would give to someone else in your situation, saying:

My voice and heart still matter.

Accepting painful truths can be difficult for anyone.

I may feel alone and separate right now, yet many others have walked in my shoes.

I am more capable of coping than I sometimes feel.

It is easy to forget that there is a difference between fighting painful facts and fighting for my health.

The fact that I tend to think more about fears of the future than how I am living right now is understandable.

Many people's actions are not consistent with their priorities.

It's always possible to have or build a meaningful life.

Emotions

Can you observe whether you're feeling disappointed, frightened, angry, regretful, resigned, and/or sad? Recall that powerful emotions are not unusual and labeling what you're feeling helps you manage those feelings. **Name it to tame it.** Hopefully, you will find it helpful to use many of the other skills presented to manage intense feelings, including the **opposite action** strategies to reverse counterproductive anxious, sad, or angry inclinations presented in Chapters 4, 5, and 6.

Distress Tolerance

If you're very agitated, you may also want to consider some of the short-term techniques presented in Chapter 4 to help your mind put you in a more comfortable place as you are trying to deal with what you have to face. **Imagery** and some of the **self-soothing** strategies from Chapter 6 may also be helpful at this time.

Cope Ahead

Many find this skill, first presented in Chapter 4, to be useful when they have to accept distressing realities. The idea is to develop a strategy to cope if what you fear is indeed true. Some consider the way they wish to live if they may not live as long as they hoped or planned. For example, one man resolved to live more fully in the present moment, paying attention to what is happening right now by noticing the beauty of nature and changing seasons. Another woman decided to try to live with more dignity, stop sweating the small stuff, and be more empathic. She wanted to leave the past behind and let go of a longtime grievance against her sister-in-law. She did realize she might have to use opposite action to get herself to act nicer to her sister-in-law! Others strive to express their fullest self or fulfill their unique role and purpose. For one man that meant more fully embracing his role as Grandpa. For one woman that meant letting her humorous side flourish. Another woman planned to nurture her creativity, spending more time with her drawing.

Let's now look at ways to focus on what is most significant to you.

Connecting to What Is Meaningful

Use wise mind to identify what is most important to you. See if you can pause to consider who or what is or has been significant and nourishing to you. Being clear about what sustains and matters to you can help you assess whether you're living the way you want to or decide what if any changes you want to make to promote the more meaningful parts of life.

Try to notice what may seem like small pieces of a mosaic that form a larger picture of what is important. A meaningful life does not require grand gestures or inspiring missions to impact the world. Meaning is very personal.

Focus on your values, beliefs, the way you wish to live, and what or who makes a difference to YOU. To assess what is most meaningful to you, ask yourself the following questions:

- Can you recall memories, relationships, places, or traditions that have made the greatest impact on you?
- Are there particular people, places, or activities that bring you joy?
- Who or what has helped you in moments of fear and doubt?
- Consider your priorities at this time.
- Do you now want to focus more or less on certain relationships?
- Do you feel differently about work/life balance?
- Is it important to you to be more loving and/or open to being loved?
- Are there people or organizations for which you feel responsible or activities that give you a sense of purpose?

- Do you especially enjoy listening to music, looking at art, or reading certain literature? Is your own creativity meaningful to you?
- Think about the sounds, sights, and smells that move you. Can you notice whether pleasures such as the gentle wind on your face, an intimate conversation, quiet time to read, or a sweet glance are significant to you?

Meaningful Relationships and Actions

Are your bonds with others the most significant part of life? Recall that social connections have been linked to better pain tolerance and survival rates. Keep in mind that it is never too late to deepen relationships that aren't all you want them to be. The interpersonal skills presented in Chapter 7 may help you express yourself and listen to another. Don't forget that supportive connections don't require a biological link. Maybe your nurturing bond comes from being part of a chosen family. Perhaps you're sustained by a relationship with a friend, neighbor, coworker, medical provider, or pet. Marsha finds the time she spends with her dog on her lap to be one of the most special parts of her day. She feels he is such a sweetheart and cherishes her morning walks with him.

Have you considered joining or getting more involved with a community, support, or therapy group? The physical and emotional link may help you feel less isolated and alone. Recall that research shows that cancer support groups improve quality of life as well as emotional and physical well-being, with some studies reporting an impact on survival rates. In addition, participation in social support, service, yoga, religious, or political groups sometimes inspires people to act on their highest values and ideals.

Making a Meaningful Difference to Others

Are you telling yourself that your life is not meaningful because you can no longer play the same roles or do the same things with others? The truth is that there are many different ways to still have a significant impact. For example, when people can no longer do certain tasks, they sometimes become mentors or advisers, teaching others. Parents who can't meet all the demands of taking care of their children can easily underestimate the value of the time and attention they are able to devote in different ways. While one mother would have preferred attending her son's soccer game, she found she could still follow the game and cheer for him watching the live-stream video. Another parent found a lot of meaning by living as fully as he could right now and modeling coping with adversity for his son. He worked with his child on a book about Daddy, including family stories, traditions, values, and wishes for the future. This father realized that the book as well as the shared time provided invaluable connections for his son.

Try not to overlook what may seem like small ways you can make a meaningful difference to others. Don't discount the effect on someone else when you speak or act kindly. At times, the smile or the warm word of encouragement, interest, or appreciation can be even more significant than the grand gesture. Are you aware of the impact you make on others living with cancer when you share your experience and wisdom?

Do your best not to underestimate the meaningful difference your physical presence, love, and attention make to your dear ones. Ultimately, the thing that matters the most is maintaining the loving bond whenever and however you are able to do so. One mother described sitting in the kitchen with her daughter and noticing the milk out on the counter and the kitchen in disarray. When she did not have the strength to even put the milk away, she decided that her priority was to find a way to touch her daughter physically and emotionally. She wisely chose to use all her energy to sit, hold out her hand, and focus on listening to her daughter.

Meaning from Giving *and* Receiving

Meaningful relationships go in two directions, loving *and* being loved. Many of us overlook the value of allowing others to give to us. Sometimes we're so busy protecting ourselves from wanting too much or feeling too needy that we may not let others get close enough to touch us. We may deprive ourselves of the significance of feeling their full love and support. What's more, we may unwittingly be robbing a dear one of the opportunity to feel loving and effective by making a difference to us.

Recall how my pride almost kept me from allowing my sister to come to the hospital. When the shoe was on the other foot, I learned a valuable lesson. A seriously unwell friend asked me to help find a pharmacy that carried a hard-to-find medication. The friend's husband was upset that she had asked me to spend so much time and effort. I was struck by her wisdom in telling him that allowing me to do something so vital to her was a sign of the depth of the friendship and that it meant a lot to me to be able to do it. A wise person knows that allowing help benefits both the giver and the receiver.

Parents can have a particularly difficult time with role reversal and allowing a child to give them something. Like Elena in Chapter 7, many don't realize how accepting help from a child can be valuable for them both. Not wanting to burden them and being concerned about the stress it may cause are understandable reactions. Yet try not to underestimate the significance for your child of being allowed to express his or her feelings for you. The ability to provide care for you can also increase your son's or daughter's self-confidence and may deepen the relationship. One mother discovered that asking her young child to read to her gave them a special shared time and was a source of great pride for her daughter. Art Buchwald's son describes how much caring for his dying father taught him about "those old-fashioned words like character, love, patience and tolerance."

Meaning from Sharing Enduring Values and Actions

Indeed, even if you expect to live a long time, it can be important to share values and traditions that can live on. When I went through the questions above to identify what was most meaningful to me, I was surprised by an early memory of going with my then young, healthy mother as she volunteered at the American Cancer Society. I hope she knows the legacy she created for me.

People who are unwell may find particular meaning in creating lasting expressions of their feelings and what is important to them. There are many different ways to try to let others know what has been most significant to you in the past, what matters now, and/or what your hopes are for the future. For example, one man wrote up the history of his company. Another man's children taped him sharing his proudest moments, life lessons, and wisdom for future generations. He talked about how he wished to be remembered. One father made a book of family traditions, values, and wishes for the future for his children.

Some express themselves creatively by making cookbooks with family recipes, photo albums of significant childhood places and events, or shell collections from treasured beach time, or by knitting, quilting, or doing other needle or woodwork, and much more. Others find that sharing art forms such as poetry, art, literature, or film with dear ones is a valuable way to communicate things that may not be expressed as easily in words.

Intangible Sources of Meaning

Meaning can also come from sources that can't be seen, heard, or touched. For many, the connection to their own heart and values is especially significant. Some find faith in themselves and valuable guidance when they bridge to their own wise mind. A belief in universal love and compassion or that all things are connected can be particularly sustaining for certain people. In times of uncertainty a link to values such as courage, loyalty, or patriotism may be inspiring.

Bringing to mind connections with others can also be nourishing. You may feel more secure and less alone by recalling an enduring bond with someone who is not physically near you right now. Can you reminisce about warm and caring experiences you shared with loved ones? Consider your link with dear ones who came before you and are a part of your life story. Some feel less alone when they think about others who have shared their cancer experience. Maybe you can make a mental picture of an individual you know or someone in literature or history that has walked the path you are on. Perhaps you find comfort thinking about a mentor or an inspiring figure, such as Nelson Mandela, or someone who represents love, such as Mother Teresa.

Meaning from Feeling a Part of Something Larger

Spirituality is a personal belief in a connection to an intangible something beyond oneself that may or may not be religious. Some individuals are sustained by feeling a part of the larger forces of the universe. They may feel nourished by being absorbed in the wonders of science or being in nature. One man found solace by hiking in the mountains. A woman we know was reassured when she could feel the breeze outside from the open window next to her bed. And as an artist, she found particular consolation in seeing the wide palettes of nature and felt more alive when she sensed a connection to life's beauty. Can you imagine looking up at the glittering stars and feeling a connection with the miraculous way they were created? Still others find the link to sources beyond themselves through yoga, meditation, psychedelics, or mystical experience.

Some individuals find a sense of purpose in working toward a greater cause. One cancer survivor described how his political activism after treatment helped him feel that he was using his energy to make a difference in the larger world after so much energy had been put into keeping him alive. Yet this may not be a time when you have the physical or emotional energy to focus on anything beyond your immediate personal concerns.

Religious Belief

Religions provide meaning and hope through shared words, actions, and beliefs. The communal prayers, texts, rituals, values, and faith in a higher power help many feel less separate and alone. Perhaps you're someone whose relationship with the divine gives you the experience of having someone or something always with you, or a loving person who loves and cares about you and is listening. Belief in God has been described as "the ultimate social support in the face of adversity." For some, religious belief offers ways to understand a puzzling world or comfort in the hope for a life after death.

For example, a woman in her late 70s with advanced cancer shared the way her faith in God helped her feel less devastated when she was given the same diagnosis as four friends who were no longer alive. She felt God would always be with her and support her. She never asked "Why me?" but felt "Why not me?" She believed whatever happened would be God's will.

Although she literally flew to Lourdes to bathe in the holy water, her prayers were not for a miracle cure but to help her accept whatever was going to happen. Accepting God's will did not mean giving up or not fighting for her health. She hopefully tried every possible medical option she could. She shared a version of a story about a man who had died in a flood to illustrate the difference between acceptance of God's will and giving up.

When the pouring rain began, the man said he had faith in God and wasn't worried. He refused to get on the boat that came to evacuate him. As the waters rose, he went up on the roof. He then sent away the helicopter that came for him. When he later got to heaven, he asked God what happened. God responded, "Didn't you see the boat and helicopter I sent for you?"

Rabbi Harold Kushner expresses a similar view: "People who pray for miracles usually don't get miracles. But people who pray for courage, for strength to bear the unbearable, for the grace to remember what they have left instead of what they have lost, very often find their prayers answered."

She felt her ability to accept what might happen was life affirming. Now, 5 years after initial diagnosis, she has been told she is cancer free. She says she is more aware of the gift of life and actively works to use whatever time she has wisely and joyfully.

Your Own Heart

Reaching for *your* sources of meaning, comfort, hope, and a sense of belonging can be extremely valuable at this time. Your solace may come from relationships with others, tangible or intangible connections to a greater force, religious traditions, and/or the higher power that fits with your beliefs. Issues of meaning, faith, and spirituality are now considered an essential element of optimal supportive care for patients with advanced cancer. Although spirituality is one of many factors, it has been linked to better immune functioning, lower risk of developing cancer, greater emotional and physical health, pain tolerance, and survival.

If you're feeling alone, doubtful, or alienated, try to keep in mind that others have felt this way. In challenging times, human and/or spiritual relationships may not always offer all we want and need. Do your best to remember that relationships aren't simply black *or* white, perfect *or* useless. It may not be in your interest to just abandon a disappointing connection. Feelings and thoughts change. Relationships may evolve. Some people are surprised to discover how much peace, strength, and solace they find in personal, spiritual, and/or communal relationships that temporarily seemed inadequate. Sometimes they renew a connection or discover a different bond.

Others may not always share your source of comfort or find it in the same way. One woman confided that she prays multiple times a day, but her otherwise very loving and supportive husband would never understand. Some prefer to express their feelings in solitude; some may want to join with others. Doubt, fear, longings, hopes, wishes, or gratitude may be expressed in prayer. Yet thoughts and feelings do not necessarily need to be directed to God or an object of worship. It is also possible to use secular readings, meditations, songs, or personal affirmations in your own words to convey what's in your heart. Significant occasions can be marked by religious ritual or secular symbolic actions such as the custom of ringing a bell at the end of chemotherapy. One man described the comfort he felt when a hospice worker had his family hold hands, share with him what had been meaningful in each of their relationships, and express their hopes for the future. Consider consulting clergy, chaplains, hospice or social workers, books, or the Internet for options to mark a moment and express your feelings in ways that can help you feel more understood and validated and less alone.

A Final Word

Living with cancer may be among the hardest things you have ever done. You may be thrown off balance. Life may seem darker. Yet you always have a choice about how you play the cards you are dealt. Even when you don't have all the control you want, your voice and heart still matter. Your actions can make a difference. You can choose to use some of the skills presented in this book.

You can do your best to honestly face what is happening. You can try to focus on the present, keeping in mind that change is constant and there is always another perspective on your situation. Coping is a balancing act, and it's possible to adjust the way you feel and think. Even when life appears dark, light and hope exist. Paying attention to your thoughts, emotions, and bodily sensations and taking steps to impact their interaction may help you handle your situation in a different way.

Even though you can't know the future, you have the option of deciding to ride the seesaw of life in the present. You can choose to live as fully and meaningfully as possible right now.

Notes

Introduction

Page 1: Studies have shown that psychosocial support for cancer patients can often improve quality of life _and_ survival rates.

Andersen, B. L., Thornton, L. M., Shapiro, C. L., Farrar, W. B., Mundy, B. L., Yang, H. C., et al. (2010). Biobehavioral, immune, and health benefits following recurrence for psychological intervention participants. *Clinical Cancer Research, 16*(12), 3270–3278.

Andersen, B. L., Yang, H. C., Farrar, W. B., Golden-Kreutz, D. M., Emery, C. F., Thornton, L. M., et al. (2008). Psychological intervention improves survival for breast cancer patients: A randomized clinical trial. *Cancer, 113*(12), 3450–3458.

Hoyt, M. A., Stanton, A. L., Bower, J. E., Thomas, K. S., Litwin, L. S., Breen, E. C., et al. (2013). Inflammatory biomarkers and emotional approach coping in men with prostate cancer. *Brain, Behavior, and Immunity, 32*, 173–179.

Jacobsen, P., & Andrykowski, M. (2015). Tertiary prevention in cancer care: Understanding and addressing the psychological dimensions of cancer during the active treatment period. *American Psychologist, 70*(2) 134–145.

Stanton, A. L., Danoff-Burg, S., Cameron, C. L., Bishop, M., Collins, C. A., Kirk, S. B., et al. (2000). Emotionally expressive coping predicts psychological and physical adjustment to breast cancer. *Journal of Consulting and Clinical Psychology, 68*(5), 875–882.

Page 1: Social and emotional treatment has not kept pace with the remarkable medical progress.

Institute of Medicine, Committee on Psyschosocial Services to Cancer Patients/Families in a Community Setting. (2008). Cancer care for the whole patient: Meeting psychosocial health needs. Washington, DC: National Academies Press.

Page 5: We can not change the cards we are dealt, just how we play the hand.

Pausch, R., & Zaslow, J. (2008). *The last lecture.* New York: Hyperion.

Chapter 1

Page 8: In a classic Memorial Sloan-Kettering study of patients' troubling symptoms, four out of the top five concerns of cancer patients were about their emotional reactions.

Portenoy, R. K., Thaler, H. T., Kornblith, A. B., Lepore, J. M., Friedlander-Klar, H., Kiyasu, E., et al. (1994). The Memorial Symptom Assessment Scale: An instrument for the evaluation of symptom prevalence, characteristics and distress. *European Journal of Cancer, 30A*(9), 1326–1336.

Page 10: Fear, sadness, and anger are considered the most common emotional responses to a cancer diagnosis.

Jacobsen, P., & Andrykowski, M. (2015). Tertiary prevention in cancer care: Understanding and addressing the psychological dimensions of cancer during the active treatment period. *American Psychologist, 70*(2), 134–145.

Moorey, S., & Greer, S. (2012). *Oxford guide to CBT for people with cancer.* Oxford, UK: Oxford University Press

Portenoy, R. K., Thaler, H. T., Kornblith, A. B., Lepore, J. M., Friedlander-Klar, H., Kiyasu, E., et al. (1994). The Memorial Symptom Assessment Scale: An instrument for the evaluation of symptom prevalence, characteristics and distress. *European Journal of Cancer, 30A*(9), 1326–1336.

Page 14: The brain is like Velcro for negative thoughts and Teflon for positive ones.

Hanson, R. (2009). *Buddha's brain: The practical neuroscience of happiness, love and wisdom.* Oakland, CA: New Harbinger.

Page 16: In wise mind, you flexibly express emotions to cope more effectively.

Westphal, M., Seivert, N. H., & Bonanno, G. A. (2010). Expressive flexibility. *Emotion, 10,* 92–100.

Chapter 2

Page 24: Research has shown that being aware of physical and emotional distress improves your ability to cope.

Levitt, J. T., Brown, T. A., Orsillo, S. M., & Barlow, D. H. (2004). The effects of acceptance versus suppression of emotion on subjective and psychophysiological response to carbon dioxide challenge in patients with panic disorder. *Behavior Therapy*, 35(4), 747–766.

Paulson, S. R., Davidson, R., Jha, A., & Kabat-Zinn, J. K. (2013). Becoming conscious: The science of mindfulness. *Annals of the New York Academy of Sciences, 1303,* 87–104.

Zeidan, F. K., Martucci, R., Kraft, N., Gordon, J., McHaffrie, J., & Coghill, R. (2011). Brain mechanisms supporting the modulation of pain by mindfulness meditation. *Journal of Neuroscience, 14,* 5540–5548.

Page 24: Mindfulness practice has been shown to help cancer patients lessen depression.

Godfrin, K. A., & van Heeringen, C. (2010). The effects of mindfulness-based cognitive therapy on recurrence of depressive episodes, mental health and quality of life: A randomized controlled study. *Behaviour Research and Therapy, 48,* 738–746.

Greeson, J. M., Smoski, M. J., Suarez, E. C., Brantley, J. G., Ekblad, A. G., & Lynch, T. R. (2015). Decreased symptoms of depression after mindfulness-based stress reduction: Potential moderating effects of religiosity, spirituality, trait mindfulness, sex, and age. *Journal of Alternative and Complementary Medicine, 21*(3), 166–174.

Gross, C. R., Kreitzer, M. J., Reily-Spong, M., Winbush, N. Y., Schomaker, E. K., & Thomas, W. (2009). Mindfulness meditation training to reduce symptom distress in transplant patients: Rationale, design, and experience with a recycled waitlist. *Clinical Trials, 6*(1),76–89.

Page 24: Decrease anxiety and stress.

Blaes, A. H., Fenner, D., Bachanova, V., Torkelson, C. J., Geller, M. A., & Hadded, T. (2016). Mindfulness-based cancer recovery in survivors recovering from chemotherapy and radiation, *Journal of Community and Supportive Oncology, 14*(8), 351–358.

Kabat-Zinn, J., Massion, A. O., Kristeller, J., Peterson, L. G., Fletcher, D. E., Pbert, L., et al. (1992). Effectiveness of a meditation-based stress reduction program in the treatment of anxiety disorders. *American Journal of Psychiatry, 149,* 936–943.

Kim, Y. H., Kim, H. J., Ahn, S. D., Seo, Y. J., & Kim, S. H. (2013). Effects of meditation on anxiety, depression, fatigue, and quality of life of women undergoing radiation therapy for breast cancer. *Complementary Therapies in Medicine, 21*(4), 379–387.

Page 24: Minimize difficulties with sleep and fatigue.

Blaes, A. H., Fenner, D., Bachanova, V., Torkelson, C. J., Geller, M. A., & Hadded, T. (2016). Mindfulness-based cancer recovery in survivors recovering from chemotherapy and radiation, *Journal of Community and Supportive Oncology*, *14*(8), 351–358.

Kim, Y. H., Kim, H. J., Ahn, S. D., Seo, Y. J., & Kim, S. H. (2013). Effects of meditation on anxiety, depression, fatigue, and quality of life of women undergoing radiation therapy for breast cancer. *Complementary Therapies in Medicine*, *21*(4), 379–387.

Page 24: Improve tolerance of physical pain.

Chiesa, A., & Serretti, A. (2011). Mindfulness-based interventions for chronic pain: A systematic review of the evidence. *Journal of Alternative and Complementary Medicine*, *17*(1), 83–93.

Zeidan, F., Martucci, K. T., Kraft, R. A., Gordon, N. S., McHaffie, J. G., & Coghills, R. C. (2011). Brain mechanisms supporting the modulation of pain by mindfulness meditation. *Journal of Neuroscience*, *31*(14), 5540–5548.

Page 24: Impact immune functioning.

Creswell, J. D., Myers, H. F., Cole, S. W., & Irwin, M. R. (2009). Mindfulness meditation training effects on CD4+ T lymphocytes in HIV-1 infected adults: A small randomized controlled trial. *Brain, Behavior, and Immunity*, *23*(2), 184–188.

Davidson, R. J., Schumacher, J. R., Muller, D., Urbanowski, F., Bonus, K., & Kabat-Zinn, J. (2003). Alterations in brain and immune function produced by mindfulness meditation. *Psychosomatic Medicine*, *65*, 564–570.

Page 24: Increase empathy/compassion.

Birnie, K., Speca, M., & Carlson, L. E. (2010). Exploring self-compassion and empathy in the context of mindfulness-based stress reduction (MBSR). *Stress and Health*, *26*, 359–371.

Chapter 3

Page 36: Suppressing emotions can get in the way of effective coping. Blocking feelings actually intensifies them.

Campbell-Sills, L., Barlow, D. H., Brown, T. A., & Hofmann S. G. (2006). Effects of suppression and acceptance on emotional responses of individuals with anxiety and mood disorders. *Behaviour Research and Therapy*, *44*, 1251–1263.

Gross, J. J., & Levenson, R. W. (1997). Hiding feelings: The acute effects of inhibiting negative and positive emotion. *Journal of Abnormal Psychology*, *106*, 95–103.

Page 36: Cancer patients who could understand, categorize, and label their emotions showed improved emotional coping and other health benefits such as lower levels of inflammation.

Hoyt, M., Stanton, A. L., Bower, J. E., Thomas, K. S., Litwin, M. S., Breen, E. C., et al. (2013). Inflammatory biomarkers and emotional approach coping in men with prostate cancer. *Brain, Behavior, and Immunity, 32,* 173–179.

Stanton, A. L., Danoff-Burg, S., Cameron, C. L., Bishop, M., Collins, C. A., & Kirk, S. B. (2000). Emotionally expressive coping predicts psychological and physical adjustment to breast cancer. *Journal of Consulting and Clinical Psychology, 68*(5), 875–882.

Stanton, A. L., & Low, C. A. (2012). Expressing emotions in stressful contexts: Benefits, moderators, and mechanisms. *Current Directions in Psychological Science, 21*(2), 124–128.

Page 37: Openly showing feeling has been found to communicate trustworthiness and increase social connection.

Boone, R. T., & Buck, R. (2003). Emotional expressivity and trustworthiness: The role of nonverbal behavior in the evolution of cooperation. *Journal of Nonverbal Behavior, 27,* 163–182.

Feinberg, M., Willer, R., Stellar, J., & Keltner, D. (2012). The virtues of gossip: Reputational information sharing as prosocial behavior. *Journal of Personality and Social Psychology, 102*(5), 1015–1030.

Mauss, I. B., Shallcross, A. J., Troy, A. S., John, O. P., Ferrer, E., Wilhelm, F. H., et al. (2011). Don't hide your happiness!: Positive emotion dissociation, social connectedness, and psychological functioning. *Journal of Personality and Social Psychology, 100*(4), 738–748.

Page 37: Physiologically this emotion, or any emotion, for that matter, lasts only for approximately 90 seconds.

Siegel, D. (2013). *Brainstorm: The power and purpose of the teenage brain.* New York: Jeremy P. Tarcher/Penguin.

Taylor, J. B. (2008). *My stroke of insight: A brain scientist's personal journey.* New York: Penguin.

Page 41: Labeling an emotion calms the central nervous system.

Badenoch, B. (2008). *Being a brain-wise therapist: A practical guide to interpersonal neurobiology.* New York: Norton.

Page 45: Slowing down the heart rate activates the parasympathetic nervous system.

Jerath, R., Edry, J. W., Barnes, V. A., & Jerath, V. (2006). Physiology of long pranayama breathing: Neural respiratory elements may provide a mechanism that explains how slow deep breathing shifts the autonomic nervous system. *Medical Hypotheses, 67*(3), 566–571.

Thayer, J. F., & Steinberg, E. (2006, November). Beyond heart rate variability: Vagal regulation of allostatic systems. *Annals of the New York Academy of Sciences, 1088*(1), 361–372.

Chapter 4

Page 48: Over 51% of cancer patients surveyed said their most important need was to cope with fear.

Breitbart, W. (2002). Spirituality and meaning in supportive care: Spirituality- and meaning-centered group psychotherapy interventions in advanced cancer. *Support Care Cancer, 10*(4), 272–280.

Page 51: Mindfulness strategies have been shown to build more resilience to stress.

Lerner, R., Zeichner, S. B., & Kibler, J. (2013). Relationship between mindfulness-based stress reduction and immune function in cancer and HIV/AIDS. *Current Oncology, 2*, 62–72.

McGonigal, K. (2015). *The upside of stress.* New York: Penguin Random House.

Page 53: A positive-thinking mantra can be an unfair burden if it implies that your natural feelings are simply the result of a bad attitude or if it leaves you blaming yourself for your medical status.

De Raeve, L. (1997). Positive thinking and moral oppression in cancer care. *European Journal of Cancer Care, 6*(4), 249–256.

Ehrenreich, B. (2009). *Bright sided: How the relentless promotion of positive thinking has undermined America.* New York: Metropolitan Books.

Petticrew, M., Bell, R., & Hunter, D. (2002, November 9). Influence of psychological coping on survival and recurrence in people with cancer: Systematic review. *BMJ, 325*(7372), 1066.

Rittenberg, C. N. (1995). Positive thinking: An unfair burden for cancer patients? *Support Care in Cancer, 3*, 37–39.

Page 54: Opposite action for fear is based on effectively proven exposure-based treatments for anxiety disorders.

Anthony, M. M., & Stein, M. B. (Eds.). (2009). *Oxford handbook of anxiety and related disorders.* New York: Oxford University Press.

Page 56: Research shows that a 20-second hug along with 10 minutes of hand-holding can lower your response to stress and anxiety.

Coan, J. A., Schaefer, H. S., & Davidson, R. J. (2006). Lending a hand: Social regulation of the neural response to threat. *Psychological Science, 17*(12), 1032–1039.

Grewen, K. M., Anderson, B. J., Girdler, S. S., & Light, K. C. (2003). Warm partner contact is related to lower cardiovascular reactivity. *Behavioral Medicine, 29*(3), 123–130.

Page 56: The most important factor in determining our response to pressure is our view of our ability to handle it.

McGonigal, K. (2015). *The upside of stress.* New York: Penguin Random House.

Page 57: The full story about stress is that it both threatens *and* challenges you.

McGonigal, K. (2015). *The upside of stress.* New York: Penguin Random House.

Page 57: When you feel stressed you work harder to solve your problems and may be motivated to reach out for help.

Buchanan, T. W., & Preston, S. D. (2014). Stress leads to prosocial action in immediate need situations. *Frontiers in Behavioral Neuroscience, 8*(5), 1–6.

Crum, A., Salovey, P., & Achor, S. (2011). Evaluating a mindset training program to unleash the enhancing nature of stress. *Academy of Management Proceedings, 1*, 1–6.

Taylor, S. E. (2006). Tend and befriend: Bio-behavioral bases of affiliation under stress. *Current Directions in Psychological Science, 15*(6), 273–277.

von Dawans, B., Fischbacher, U., Kirschbaum, C., Fehr, E., & Heinrichs, M. (2012). The social dimension of stress reactivity: Acute stress increases prosocial behavior in humans. *Psychological Science, 23*(6), 651–660.

Page 58: Research shows that a fuller and more balanced view that considers both the upside and downside of stress empowers people to take control of how they respond.

Crum, A. J., Akinola, M., Martin, A., & Fath, S. (2017). The role of stress mindset in shaping cognitive, emotional, and physiological responses to challenging and threatening stress, *Anxiety, Stress, and Coping, 30*(4), 379–395.

Crum, A. J., Corbin, W. R., Brownell, K. D., & Salovey, P. (2011). Mind over milkshakes: Mindsets, not just nutrients, determine ghrelin response. *Health Psychology, 30*(4), 424–429.

Crum, A. J., & Langer, E. J. (2007). Mind-set matters: Exercise and the placebo effect. *Psychological Science, 18*(2), 165–171.

Page 58: People who see the challenge as well as the threat of stress have been shown to be more likely to trust themselves to handle the situation and rise to the challenge. Their resilience actually increases.

Aerni, A., Traber, R., Hock, C., Roozendaal, B., Schelling, G., Papassotiropoulos, A., et al. (2004). Low-dose cortisol for symptoms of posttraumatic stress disorder. *American Journal of Psychiatry, 161*(8), 1488–1490.

Jamieson, J. P., Mendes, W. B., & Nock, M. K. (2013). The power of reappraisal. *Current Directions in Psychological Science, 22*, 51–56.

Keller, A., Litzelman K., Wisk, L. E., Maddox, T., Cheng, E. R., & Creswell, P. D. (2011). Does the perception that stress affects health matter? The association with health and mortality. *Health Psychology, 31*(5), 677–684.

Page 62: Up to 80% of cancer patients have sleep problems during treatment. Sleep disruption may come from medication and/or stress and anxiety.

Carlson, L. E., & Garland, S. N. (2005). Impact of mindfulness-based stress reduction (MBSR) on sleep, mood, stress, and fatigue symptoms in cancer outpatients. *International Journal of Behavioral Medicine, 12*(4), 278–285.

Savard, J., & Morin, C. M. (2001). Insomnia in the context of cancer: A review of a neglected problem. *Journal of Clinical Oncology, 19*(3), 895–908.

Page 62: Watch out for middle-of-the-night thinking, when worries may seem even more catastrophic than in the daytime.

Harvery, A. G., & Greenall, E. (2003, March). Catastrophic worry in primary insomnia. *Experimental Psychiatry, 34*(1), 11–23.

Chapter 5

Page 64: Sadness can facilitate constructive grief.

Bonanno, G. A. (2009). *The other side of sadness: What the new science of bereavement tells us about life after loss.* New York: Basic Books.

Bonanno, G. A., Goorin, L., & Coifman, K. G. (2008). Sadness and grief. In M. Lewis, J. M. Haviland-Jones, & L. F. Barrett (Eds.), *Handbook of emotions* (3rd ed., pp. 797–810). New York: Guilford Press.

Page 64: Studies show sad people become more self-perceptive.

Bodenhausen, G. V., Sheppard, L. A., & Kramer, G. P. (1994). Negative affect and social judgment: The differential impact of anger and sadness. *European Journal of Social Psychology, 24*, 45–62.

Page 64: When people feel sad, they look sad. Their appearance elicits sympathy and sends a compelling message that connection and support are needed.

Bonanno, G. A., & Keltner, D. (1997). Facial expressions of emotion and the course of conjugal bereavement. *Journal of Abnormal Psychology, 106,* 126–137.

Page 65: Research shows that sorrow also helps build compassion and empathy. Sad people sometimes become more thoughtful and less biased in their perceptions of others.

Eisenberg, N., Fabes, R., Miller, P., Fultz, J., Shell, R., Mathy, R. M., et al. (1989). Relation of sympathy and distress to prosocial behavior: A multimethod study. *Journal of Personality and Social Psychology, 57,* 55–66.

Page 67: Studies show that people using mindfulness skills often advance more quickly through the initial stages of mourning and demonstrate significant reductions in depression and anxiety.

Sagula, D., & Rice, K. (2004). The effectiveness of mindfulness training on the grieving process and emotional well-being of chronic pain patients. *Journal of Clinical Psychology in Medical Settings, 11*(4), 333–342.

Page 67: Sad people can make negative judgments and assumptions about themselves, their coping, and their relationships.

Gilbert, P. (2009). *Overcoming depression.* New York: Basic Books.

Nezu, A., Nezu, C., & D'Zurilla, T. (2007). *Solving life's problems: A 5-step guide to enhanced well-being.* New York: Springer.

Nezu, A., Nezu, C., & D'Zurilla, T. (2012). *Problem-solving therapy: A treatment manual.* New York: Springer.

Nezu, A., Nezu, C., Friedman, S., Faddis, S., & Houts, P. (1999). *Helping cancer patients cope: A problem-solving approach.* Washington, DC: American Psychological Association Press.

Page 68: Sadness is part of a bigger picture that includes the opposite view

Stroebe, M., & Schut, H. (1999). The dual process model of coping with bereavement: Rationale and description. *Death Studies, 23*(3), 197–224.

Page 69: A fuller, balanced perspective fosters resilience. What's more, building up positive feelings can reduce the likelihood of depression and strengthen the immune system.

Bono, J., Glomb, T., Shen, W., Kim, E., & Koch, A. (2013). Building positive resources: Effects of positive events and positive reflection on work stress and health. *Academy of Management Journal, 56*(6), 1–27.

Davidson, R. J., Kabat-Zinn, J., Schumacher, M., Rosenkranz, D., Muller,

S. Santorelli, F., et al. (2003). Alterations in brain and immune function produced by mindfulness mediation. *Psychosomatic Medicine, 65*(5), 64–70.

Page 70: Research shows that at least trying to acknowledge any blessing may be worth your while.

Emmons, R. A., & McCullough, M. E. (2003). Counting blessings versus burdens: An experimental investigation of gratitude and subjective well-being in daily life. *Journal of Personality and Social Psychology, 84,* 377–389.

Page 72: Consider trying a breathing strategy called Ha breath.

Brown, R., & Gerbarg, P. (2012). *The healing power of the breath: Simple techniques to reduce stress and anxiety, enhance concentration, and balance your emotions.* Boston: Shambhala.

Page 73: Humor helps to make grief bearable and has been reported to boost mood, strengthen immune system functioning, diminish pain, and protect against damaging effects of stress. Sincere laughing and smiling are contagious and encourage more pleasant connections with others.

Bonanno, G. A. (2009). *The other side of sadness: What the new science of bereavement tells us about life after loss.* New York: Basic Books, page 37.

Page 73: Research shows that cracking a grin when the chips are down improves long-term coping.

Ibid, page 38.

Page 73: The more grieving people laughed and smiled in the early months of a loss, the better their mental health was over the next two years

Ibid, page 646.

Page 74: Mastery has been shown to increase resistance to being depressed.

Diener, E., & Seligman, M. E. P. (2002). Very happy people. *Psychological Science, 13*(1), 81–84.

Page 75: Writing about joyful experiences enhances positive mood.

Frattaroli, J. (2006). Experimental disclosure and its moderators: A meta-analysis. *Psychological Bulletin, 132,* 823–865.

Low, C. A., Stanton, A. L., & Danoff-Burg, S. (2006). Expressive disclosure and benefit finding among breast cancer patients: Mechanisms for positive health effects. *Health Psychology, 25*(2), 181–189.

Pennebaker, J. W., & Smyth, J. M. (2016). *Opening up by writing it down: How expressive writing improves health and eases emotional pain.* New York: Guilford Press.

Smyth, J. M. (1998). Written emotional expression: Effect sizes, outcome types, and moderating variables. *Journal of Consulting and Clinical Psychology, 66*, 174–184.

Page 75: The more people feel like they are helping others, the less depressed they feel.

Cristea, I. A., Legge, E., Prosperi, M., Guazzelli, M., David, D., & Gentili, C. (2014). Moderating effects of empathic concern and personal distress on the emotional reactions of disaster volunteers. *Disasters, 8*(4), 740–752.

Grant, A. M., & Sonnentag, S. (2010). Doing good buffers against feeling bad: Prosocial impact compensates for negative task and self-evaluations. *Organizational Behavior and Human Decision Processes, 111*, 13–22.

Sullivan, G. B., & Sullivan, M. J. (1997). Promoting wellness in cardiac rehabilitation: Exploring the role of altruism. *Journal of Cardiovascular Nursing, 11*(3), 43–52.

Chapter 6

Page 77: Intense hostility may endanger relationships or leave you feeling out of control or ashamed.

Burns, J. W., Higdon, L. J., Mullen, J. T., Lansky, D., & Wei, J. M. (1999). Relationships among patient hostility, anger expression, depression, and the working alliance in a work hardening program. *Annals of Behavioral Medicine, 21*(1), 77–82.

Page 77: Anger can impact the immune system or worsen pain.

Burns, J. W., Johnson, B. J., Devine, J., Mahoney, N., & Pawl, R. (1998). Anger management style and the prediction of treatment outcome among male and female chronic pain patients. *Behavioral Research Therapy, 36*, 1051–1062.

Greenwood, K., Thurston, R., Rumble, M., Waters, S. J., & Keefe, F. J. (2003). Anger and persistent pain: Current status and future directions. *Pain, 103*(1), 1–5.

Hatch, J. P., Schoenfeld, L. S., Boutros, N. N., Seleshi, E., Moore, M. A., & Cyr-Provost, M. (1991). Anger and hostility in tension-type headache. *Headache, 31*, 302–304.

Okifuji, A., Turk, D. C., & Curran, S. L. (1999). Anger in chronic pain:

Investigations of anger targets and intensity. *Journal of Psychosomatic Research, 47*(1), 1–12.

Page 79: When you ignore feelings, pain may sometimes be more severe, you may be more upset, or relationships may be compromised.

Duckro, P. N., Chibnall, J. T., & Tomazic, T. J. (1995). Anger, depression, and disability: A path analysis of relationships in a sample of chronic posttraumatic headache patients. *Headache, 3*(5), 7–9.

Kerns, R. D., Rosenberg, R., & Jacob, M. C. (1994). Anger expression and chronic pain. *Journal of Behavioral Medicine, 17,* 57–67.

Tschannen, T. A., Duckro, P. N., Margolis, R. B., Tomazic, T. J. (1992). The relationship of anger, depression, and perceived disability among headache patients. *Headache, 32,* 501–503.

Page 79: Mere anticipation of pain was enough to provoke anger in healthy individuals.

Berkowitz, L., & Thomas, P. (1987). Pain expectation, negative affect, and angry aggression. *Motivational Emotion, 11,* 183–193.

Page 81: Even a gentle walk can sometimes help you feel and think differently.

Carlson, L., & Speca, M. (2010). *Mindfulness-based cancer recovery: A step-by-step MBSR approach to help you cope with treatment and reclaim your life.* Oakland, CA: New Harbinger.

Page 84: Imagery has been shown to help cancer patients tolerate pain and other distressing situations.

Baider, L., Uziely, B., & Kaplan De-Nour, A. (1994). Progressive muscle relaxation and guided imagery in cancer patients. *General Hospital Psychiatry, 16,* 340–347.

Kwekkeboom, K. L., Kneip, J., & Pearson, L. (2003). A pilot study to predict success with guided imagery for cancer pain. *Pain Management Nursing, 4*(3), 112–123.

Lang, E. V., Ward, C., & Laser, E. (2010). Effect of team training on patients' ability to complete MRI examinations. *Academic Radiology, 17,* 18–23.

Page 87: Research has shown that self-compassion actually strengthens and motivates one to be proactive.

Neff, K. D., & Dahm, K. A. (2015). Self-compassion: What it is, what it does, and how it relates to mindfulness. In B. Ostafin, M. Robinson, & B. Meier (Eds.), *Handbook of mindfulness and self-regulation.* New York: Springer.

Page 87: There is little consistent evidence that a mindset such as a fighting spirit, hopelessness, helplessness, denial or avoidance impacts cancer survival or recurrence.

Petticrew, M., Bell, R., & Hunter, D. (2002). Influence of psychological coping on survival and recurrence in people with cancer: Systematic review. *BMJ, 325*(7372), 1066.

Page 88: Self-compassion has been shown to be effective in reducing both anger and the severity of pain. It can benefit people in chronic pain even in the absence of other pain management. It can also improve psychological well-being by decreasing anxiety, depression, and stress and increasing the capacity to accept pain.

Carson, J. W., Keefe, F. J., Lynch, T. R. Carson, K. M., Goli, V., Fras, A. M., et al. (2005). Loving-kindness meditation for chronic low back pain: Results from a pilot trial. *Journal of Holistic Nursing, 23*, 287–304.

Chapin, H. L., Darnall, B. D., Seppala, E. M., Doty, J. R., Hah, J. M., & Mackey, S. C. (2014). Pilot study of a compassion meditation intervention in chronic pain. *Journal of Compassionate Health Care, 1*(4).

Gilbert, P., McEwan, K., Catarino, F., & Baiao, R. (2014). Fears of compassion in a depressed population: Implication for psychotherapy. *Journal of Depression and Anxiety, S2*(1).

Hofmann, S. G., Grossman, P., & Hinton, D. E. (2011). Loving-kindness and compassion meditation: Potential for psychological intervention. *Clinical Psychology Review, 31*(7), 1126–1132.

Hooria, J., Jinpa, G. T., McGonigal, K., Rosenberg, E. K., Finkelstein, J., Simon-Thomas, E., et al. (2013). Enhancing compassion: A randomized controlled trial of a compassion cultivation training program. *Journal of Happiness Studies, 14*(4), 1113–1126.

Hutcherson, C. A., Seppala, E. M., & Gross, J. J. (2008). Loving kindness meditation increases social connectedness. *Emotion, 8*(5), 720–724.

Page 88: People who recognize the universality of their feelings and their common humanity, and remember that others are also suffering, have been found to be happier, more resilient, and more satisfied with life.

McGonigal, K. (2015). *The upside of stress.* New York: Penguin Random House.

Page 88: To use compassionate self-talk.

Portions of the self-talk adapted from Bernhard, T. (2010). *How to be sick: A Buddhist-inspired guide for the chronically ill and their caregivers.* Somerville, MA: Wisdom.

Chapter 7

Page 91: Your connections to others can impact life with cancer.

Deckx, L., den Akker, M., & Buntinx, F. (2014). Risk factors for loneliness in patients with cancer: A systematic literature review and meta-analysis. *European Journal of Oncology Nursing, 18*(5), 466–477.

Guntupalli, S., & Karinch, M. (2017). *Sex and cancer: Intimacy, romance, and love after diagnosis and treatment.* New York: Rowman & Littlefield.

Rokach, A., Findler, L., Chin, J., Lev, S., & Kollender, Y. (2013). Cancer patients, their caregivers, and coping with loneliness. *Psychology, Health and Medicine, 18*(2), 135–144.

Wells, M. (2008). The loneliness of cancer. *European Journal of Oncology Nursing, 12,* 410–411.

Page 91: While some worry that cancer might strain relationships, it also has the power to deepen and enhance them.

Manne, S., Ostroff, J., Winkel, G., Goldstein, L., Fox, K., & Grana, G. (2004). Posttraumatic growth after breast cancer: Patient, partner, and couple perspectives. *Psychosomatic Medicine, 66,* 442–454.

Tedeschi, R., & Calhoun, L. (2004) Posttraumatic growth: Conceptual foundations and empirical evidence. *Psychological Inquiry, 15*(1).

Page 92: Young people can find it particularly difficult to feel cut off from the normal sense of belonging and community.

Kelly, D., Pearce, S., & Mullhall, A. (2004). Being in the same boat: Ethnographic insights into an adolescent cancer unit. *International Journal of Nursing Studies, 41,* 847–857.

Page 98: In the face of crisis some people find previously untapped reservoirs of strength.

Tedeschi, R., & Calhoun, L. (2004). Posttraumatic growth: Conceptual foundations and empirical evidence. *Psychological Inquiry, 15*(1).

Page 99: Cancer-specific support groups can minimize isolation, and psychosocial support has been shown to impact cancer patients' quality of life and survival rates. Other studies link social connections to pain toleration.

Andersen, B. L., Thornton, L. M., Shapiro, C. L., Farrar, W. B., Mundy, B. L., Yang, H. C., et al. (2010). Biobehavioral, immune, and health benefits following recurrence for psychological intervention participants. *Clinical Cancer Research, 16*(12), 3270–3278.

Andersen, B. L., Yang, H. C., Farrar, W. B., Golden-Kreutz, D. M., Emery, C. F.,

Thornton, L. M., et al. (2008). Psychological intervention improves survival for breast cancer patients: A randomized clinical trial. *Cancer, 113,* 3450–3458.

Guo, Z., Tang, H.-Y., Tang, H. L., Tan, S.-K., Feng, K.-H., Huang, Y.-C., et al. (2013). The benefits of psychosocial interventions for cancer patients undergoing radiotherapy. *Health Quality of Life Outcomes, 11*(1), 121.

House, J. S., Landis, K. R., & Umberson, D. (1988). Social relationships and health. *Science, 241,* 540–554.

House, J. S., Robbins, C., & Metzner, H. L. (1982). The association of social relationships and activities with mortality: Prospective evidence from the Tecumseh Community Health study. *American Journal of Epidemiology, 116,* 123–140.

Pinquarta, M., & Duberstein, P. (2010). Associations of social networks with cancer mortality: A meta-analysis. *Critical Reviews in Oncology/Hematology, 75*(2), 122–137.

Chapter 8

Page 108: A supportive relationship with a physician has been shown to significantly impact a patient's emotional state.

Meyerowitz, B. (1980). Psychosocial correlates of breast cancer and its treatments. *Psychological Bulletin, 87*(1), 108–131.

Page 111: Could his doctor be trying to protect him as physicians trying to be sensitive can sometimes do?

Gawande, A. (2010, July 26). Letting go: What should medicine do when it can't save your life? *New Yorker.*

Page 116: Cancer may also affect how you relate to those you work with in the community or workplace.

Baxter, M. F., Newman, R., Longpré, S. M., & Polo, K. M. (2017). Occupational therapy's role in cancer survivorship as a chronic condition. *American Journal of Occupational Therapy, 71*(3).

Page 117: Mild cognitive changes sometimes referred to as "chemo brain" are common and usually subside.

Ahles, T. A., & Root, J. C. (2018). Cognitive effects of cancer and cancer treatments. *Annual Review of Clinical Psychology, 14*(5), 425–451.

Boykoff, N., Moieni, M., & Subramanian, S. K. (2009). Confronting chemo brain: An in-depth look at survivors' reports of impact on work, social networks, and health care response. *Journal of Cancer Survivorship, 3,* 223–232.

Janselins, M. C., Kesler, S. R., Ahles, T. A., & Morrow, G. R. (2014). Prevalence, mechanisms, and management of cancer-related cognitive impairment. *International Review of Psychiatry, 26*(1), 102–111.

Page 120: Understandably, economic insecurity can shake one's sense of control.

Chou, E. Y., Bidhan, P. L., & Galinsky, A. D. (2016). Economic insecurity increases physical pain. *Psychological Science, 27,* 443–454.

Page 120: Ways others have dealt with attention or memory difficulties.

Newman, R. (2020). Cancer related cognitive impairment. In B. Braveman & R. Newman (Eds.), *Cancer and occupational therapy: Enabling occupational performance and participation across the lifespan.* Bethesda, MD: AOTA Press.

Chapter 9

Page 124: Research has shown that people with advanced cancer who focused their energy on what was most meaningful to them felt less hopeless and depressed.

Brady, M. J., Peterman, A. H., Fitchett, G., Mo, M., & Cella, D. (1999). A case of including spirituality in quality of life measurement in oncology. *Psycho-oncology, 8,* 417–428.

Breitbart, W., & Heller, K. S. (2003). Reframing hope: Meaning-centered care for patients near the end of life. *Journal of Palliative Medicine, 6,* 979–988.

Breitbart, W., Rosenfeld, B., Pessin, H., Kaim, M., Funesti-Esch, J., Galietta, M., et al. (2000). Depression, hopelessness, and desire for hastened death in terminally ill cancer patients. *Journal of American Medical Association, 284,* 2907–2911.

McClain, C., Rosenfeld, B., & Breitbart, W. (2003). The effect of spiritual well-being on end-of-life despair in terminally ill cancer patients. *Lancet, 361,* 1603–1607.

Nelson, C., Rosenfeld, B., Breitbart, W., & Galietta, M. (2002). Spirituality, depression and religion in the terminally ill. *Psychosomatics, 43,* 213–220.

Page 131: Identify what is most important to you.

Adapted from Breitbart, W., & Heller, K. S. (2003). Reframing hope: Meaning-centered care for patients near the end of life. *Journal of Palliative Medicine, 6,* 979–988.

Page 134: Art Buchwald's son describes how much caring for his dying father taught him about "those old-fashioned words like character, love, patience and tolerance."

Strupp, J. (2007, January 19). Art Buchwald's son calls past year "a rollercoaster." *Editor and Publisher.*

Page 135: You may feel more secure and less alone by recalling an enduring bond with someone who is not physically near you right now.

Cacioppo, J., & Patrick, W. (2008). *Loneliness: Human nature and the need for human connection.* New York: Norton.

Page 136: Still others find the link to sources beyond themselves through yoga, meditation, psychedelics, or mystical experience.

Pollan, M. (2018). *How to change your mind: What the new science of psychedelics teaches us about consciousness, dying, addiction, depression and transcendence.* New York: Penguin Press.

Page 137: "People who pray for miracles usually don't get miracles. But people who pray for courage, for strength to bear the unbearable, for the grace to remember what they have left instead of what they have lost, very often find their prayers answered."

Kushner, H. (1981). *When bad things happen to good people.* New York: Random House.

Page 137: Issues of meaning, faith, and spirituality are now considered an essential element of optimal supportive care for patients with advanced cancer.

Brady, M. J., Peterman, A. H., Fitchett, G., Mo, M., & Cella, D. (1999). A case of including spirituality in quality of life measurement in oncology. *Psychooncology, 8,* 417–428.

Breitbart, W. (2002). Spirituality and meaning in supportive care: Spirituality- and meaning-centered group psychotherapy interventions in advanced cancer. *Support Care Cancer, 10*(4), 272–280.

Page 137: Although spirituality is one of many factors, it has been linked to better immune functioning, lower risk of developing cancer, greater emotional and physical health, pain tolerance, and survival.

Brady, M. J., Peterman, A. H., Fitchett, G., Mo, M., & Cella, D. (1999). A case of including spirituality in quality of life measurement in oncology. *Psychooncology, 8,* 417–428.

Breitbart, W. (2002). Spirituality and meaning in supportive care: Spirituality- and meaning-centered group psychotherapy interventions in advanced cancer. *Support Care Cancer, 10*(4), 272–280.

Marchant, J. (2016). *Cure: A journey into the science of mind over body.* New York: Penguin Random House.

Nicholson, A., Rose, R., & Bobak, M. (2009). Association between attendance at religious services and self-reported health in 22 European countries. *Social Science and Medicine, 69,* 519–528.

Page 137: Some people are surprised to discover how much peace, strength, and solace they find in personal, spiritual, and/or communal relationships that temporarily seemed inadequate. Sometimes they renew a connection and discover a different bond.

Personal communication with Rabbi Edythe Held Mencher, LCSW.

Page 138: Thoughts and feelings do not necessarily need to be directed to God or an object of worship. It is also possible to use secular readings, meditations, songs, or personal affirmations in your own words to convey what's in your heart.

Personal communication with Rabbi Edythe Held Mencher, LCSW.

Index

Note. *f* following a page number indicates a figure.

About the Authors

Elizabeth Cohn Stuntz, LCSW, a psychotherapist in private practice in Mamaroneck, New York, is a cancer survivor and a Zen student. After many years of involvement with services for people with cancer and their loved ones, she developed a program of coping skills based on DBT. She serves on the faculty of the Westchester Center for Psychoanalysis and Psychotherapy.

Marsha M. Linehan, PhD, ABPP, the developer of DBT, is Professor Emeritus of Psychology and Director Emeritus of the Behavioral Research and Therapy Clinics at the University of Washington. Dr. Linehan's contributions to clinical psychology research have been recognized with numerous prestigious awards. In 2018, she was featured in a special issue of *Time* magazine, "Great Scientists: The Geniuses and Visionaries Who Transformed Our World." She is a Zen master.